Ketogenic Diet

The Ultimate Fat Burning Cookbook

©Maya Lyon

Forward

I would like to thank you for purchasing "The Ketogenic Diet: The Ultimate Fat Burning Cookbook" and congratulate you for taking the steps to improve your health and wellbeing.

To say that the Ketogenic diet is life-changing would be an understatement. Following the Ketogenic diet will allow you take control of your health and the benefits that will spill over to all parts of your life. Of course you can expect to see physical changes like definite weight loss and an increase in stamina and strength, and just generally feeling more comfortable in your own skin.

This book will use a step-wise approach to take you through the Ketogenic journey and further beyond into the practical application of making healthy and super tasty recipes. The Ketogenic diet expounds on a practical and sustainable way to nourish our bodies to maintain lifelong health, physical performance and overall wellness.

As you embark on this health journey, I hope it leads you to a life of pure health bliss and vitality as it has for so many Ketogenic devotees."

Table of Contents

5

Chapter 1

Overview of the Ketogenic Diet

What is it?

Human metabolism has not adapted to our standard western diet.

Our bodies have not evolved to process modern-day carbohydrate rich foodstuffs.

Our ancient ancestors used to hunt for meals, and would often go for days, if not weeks without food. When food became scarce, the body would switch from using food as its main energy source and utilize fat reserves instead. In our day and age food is far more plentiful, and unfortunately the food nowadays is rich in empty calorie carbohydrates which is quickly stored as fat if not used.

The concept of the ketogenic diet takes advantage of your body's natural systems that utilize fat for fuel instead of carbs. This high fat, low carb diet that will put your body in a state of ketosis, exactly what our lean and healthy ancestors experienced. The process of ketosis will allow ketones (converted fats) to be produced in your liver and these will be your primary source of energy, resulting in weight loss.

Our bodies usually use glucose and insulin for energy and this is acquired through foods that contain carbohydrates. However on the ketogenic diet there is a very low intake of carbohydrates, thus the body turns to fats as its primary source of fuel, as paraphrased in the first paragraph. On a normal basis we would consume various foods that contain carbohydrates and these foods help to sustain our energy for each day. However for some of us consuming too many carbohydrates usually ends up in weight gain if we do not burn the excess calories off with exercise. Not to mention the chronic diseases of lifestyle such as diabetes which often result from high carbohydrate diets. If you happen to be diabetic or struggle with eating a healthy amount of carbohydrates then this diet is the perfect solution.

Now just to be clear as to what happens on the keto diet, you will be eating high levels of fat and low levels of carbohydrates. Do not be alarmed by this as the fats will not be acting as a secondary source of energy in this diet but as the main source thus all fats consumed will be used up by the body. But why would you eat more fats if you want to be healthier you may ask. I will explain a bit more.

Eating higher levels of fats and lower levels of carbs will put your body in a state of ketosis which will trick your body into thinking it is starving. In this 'starvation' mode your body will seek out the greatest source of energy to maintain its self, which in this case will be fats. Be reassured you won't actually be starving nor will you be gaining weight from the increased levels of fat. Your body will simply adapt to this new way and start to target the only source of energy that seems viable, fats. Don't be puzzled, that was just a brief introduction into this intriguing diet; let's us learn a bit more.

Tips for Starting the Keto Journey

The main thing about the ketogenic diet is that you have to plan ahead; this is why the ketogenic diet is seen as a lifestyle rather than a diet. Planning ahead will ensure that you always have enough to eat and so that your journey will be as smooth and organized as possible. It also ensures that you will have foods that will help keep your body in 'ketosis'. Firstly it depends on how soon you intend to put your body in 'ketosis'. Since this is done through lowering carbs and increasing fats then then the less carbs and more fats you intake will decide how soon this is achieved. What exactly are you going to eat? On most diets about 20g of carbohydrates are required, however on the keto diet you will consuming only about 15g or less. You will have an example further on in this book so you can have a clearer understanding.

The following tips will help to make going into the keto diet much easier and I certainly hope all of them will help.

- *Get rid of all high carb foods in your pantry-* In order to lessen temptation and to make sure you start your diet on a clean slate. Throw out all high carb foods, acceptable carbs will be discussed further on in the book.
- *Restock your kitchen-* After getting rid of all the 'bad' stuff, replace them with all the low carb goodies you will need. There is really no need for 'special' foods when doing this. You will simply be buying whole foods and less processed food.
- *Learn to measure your food in net carbs-* In case you are not familiar with net carbs, it is very simple to understand. The net carbs in your food is the dietary carb minus the fiber. Let us make this a little easier by using an example. If broccoli has 6g

of carbs per cup and there are 2g of fiber. We simply deduct 2g from 6g which gives us 4g; this is the net carb.

- *Stick to 20g of carbs or less daily*- In order to get the body into ketosis and keep it there, you have to eat as little carbohydrates as possible. This plays an intricate role in the ketogenic diet and this has to be precisely done to avoid hampering progress. Always double and triple check to make sure you are not having too many carbohydrates. Your daily intake of carbs should only be 5-10% of all meals.

- *Eat lots of vegetables*- You can never go wrong when you choose vegetables on the ketogenic diet. However be sure to stick to those vegetables that are low carb. Eating vegetables will also fill you up and help you to eat less protein which is also a key factor in the ketogenic diet.

- *Do not have too much protein*- Protein intake promotes increases in your insulin levels, the higher your insulin levels the less likely you are to lose weight. Special attention must be paid to this so that one may not be deterred by slow progress. The protein intake should account for around 20-25% of the meals daily.

- *Fats should account for 65% of meals*- Though fats will be your main source of energy and the basis on which you will make each meal. Do not overdo it but try not to miss your target either. You can use whatever method you prefer that can help to calculate this.

- *Avoid cheating*- You may be tempted to cheat on your diet but this should be totally avoided as you can easily throw your body out of ketosis and your hard earned progress will be hampered. You simply have to accept that the ketogenic diet is a long term commitment that your body will thank you for. You simply don't want to betray yourself by cheating on it.

- **Drink lots of water-** Drinking water in any case does wonders for the body and on this diet it is no different. You will need lots of water to rehydrate your body because the changes will flush your body. There may be an increase in urination as your body flushes excess water that was once retained from eating carbohydrates. You can stick to 8 glasses a day and have more if you feel it is necessary.

- **You will be spending more time in the kitchen-** This may not be the highlight of this diet but in order to get the fantastic results that the ketogenic diet offers, you will have to spend a bit of time in the kitchen so get those aprons on and get cooking. You can even prepare some meals that you can take on the go so as to avoid having to grab fast food. Preparing your own food ensures that you know exactly what you are eating.

- **Plan your meals-** It's all about planning on the keto diet, the more you plan for your meals the less likely you are to fall into the old habit of having high carb foods. Make a shopping list when you head to the store and try your best to stick to it.

- **Consider taking supplements-** Though not necessary, you may consider taking supplements, these can help suppress cravings for sugar especially in the initial start of the keto diet.

- **Read up as much as you can before starting the diet-** Since the keto diet is one of those diets that you have to be committed to for a long time, it is best to read up about the diet to make sure you know exactly what is expected and to make sure that you can handle the new changes. You should also check with your physician to make sure this is the right kind of diet for you as some persons may be exempt.

- *Know the difference between ketoacidosis and ketosis-* These two terms will certainly pop up whenever looking into the ketogenic diet. Some physicians may not be equipped with the proper knowledge so it is best that you find out the difference between these terms especially as to avoid misconceptions about the ketogenic diet.
- *Avoid exercising in the first 3 weeks-* This is one of those diets that you will really have no need to do excessive exercise. As your body undergoes the new dietary changes your body may show some signs that may not be conducive to exercise. No need to worry even without exercise you will certainly be able to tell the difference in those first 3 weeks. This is also great for extremely overweight persons are even disabled individuals.
- *Take pictures-* . In the first month you may not even believe how much weight you will lose but by taking pictures you will be able to visually see the changes. Taking pictures throughout the keto journey will be motivation to continue on the diet

Exercise

You may have read or heard that you don't need exercise to lose weight. Most diets always promote exercise to make the dieting more rewarding however on the keto diet exercising is optional. So if you are unable to exercise for whatever reason you will still be able to get all the weight loss benefits.

If you are able to exercise and would like to continue doing so then that's even better news for you as the weight loss process is greater on the keto diet than other low fat diets. Since your main source of energy is coming from fats your body will be targeting all available fat sources, this includes those eaten and those within the body. This is why you can lose weight whether or not you choose to exercise however exercising can help you to keep toned and can help with muscle gain. Exercising is really up to you-you decide.

In the case you choose exercise then you should start with light exercises such as walking or swimming, this can be done for 30 minutes about 3 days per week. As you get fit you can increase the intensity and length of your workouts as you see it fit. Exercising does not affect the rate of ketosis; your food decides on that however exercise promotes speedy weight loss.

For athletes or very active person the exercise approach will be different as initially the body will not be able to perform vigorous exercises. An active person may have to take on the cyclical keto diet wherein you have lots of carbohydrates on the weekend and low carb during the week.

Wow we have really covered a lot so far and we have so much more to cover but I certainly hope that you have a much clearer understanding going forward. I am pretty sure you may have much more unanswered questions. Maybe you heard some stories that may have you reconsidering the keto experience. We will next take a look into misconceptions, pros and cons and much more.

Demolishing myths about the keto diet

As with any diet there are naysayers and persons with no experience or knowledge of the diet that may circulate myths about the diet. If you have heard or read any of these misconceptions then this highlight will be more than helpful.

1.   **The high fat intake on the keto diet will lead to heart attacks**

With the term high fat, most persons have formulated this misconception and it is by far the biggest misconception as it relates to the keto diet; let us demolish this notion. Since fat is the source of energy it is also being used up by the body constantly so the chances of excess fat being stored is not likely. If the keto diet is compared to a 'regular' diet wherein more carbs are being ingested then the chances of weight loss is actually slower on a regular diet and there is a greater possibility that excess fat can be stored since the body would be targeting carbs for energy. Since ketosis is tricking the body into thinking it is starving then the cells are working to eat up all the fat which is the most viable source to keep them going. The high fat content of the keto diet is not in any way likely to suddenly clog arteries or give you a heart attack as all fat is being used up by the body.

2.   **Eating little carbs damages the kidneys**

Most low carb diets are high in protein which has been linked to kidney issues however the keto diet requires moderate protein intake so no need to worry about any kidney damage. You will possibly be having no more protein than you usually have.

3.   **Putting your body in ketosis is dangerous**

This misconception is from a lack of understanding of the two terms that always come up when the ketogenic diet is mentioned. Ketosis is sometimes confused with ketoacidosis. Ketoacidosis is when the body produces abnormal amounts of ketones and this usually takes place in an uncontrolled situation. Ketosis on the other hand is usually controlled and is the process wherein the body releases ketones because of the low carb, high fat intake. Ketosis promotes the release of ketones

15

in a controlled way whereas ketoacidosis can only occur when insulin is nonexistent and there is no way to control ketones. Ketosis is only dangerous to persons with type 1 diabetes.

These myths can be taken into consideration if you have a pre-existing kidney condition or if you have type 1 diabetes. The ketogenic diet is more appropriate for persons with type 2 diabetes. Please consult your doctor before embarking on any diet and to discuss any issues you may have before doing the keto diet.

Side effects

You will certainly all the benefits that you will receive from being on the ketogenic diet. You will see progress and you will be pleased with them, your body will be better on the inside and out. However as with any diet there are a few side effects that you may face.

1. **Leg Cramps**

In the early phase of the keto journey some persons have reported having leg cramps especially during the night time. This is as a result of the lack of potassium that the body is getting and may be rectified through supplements.

2. **Headaches/ Dizziness**

This is the most common side effect. You may get some headaches or feel light headed initially as you start the keto diet. This is as a result of your body reacting to changes in sugar. Also if you are a caffeine drinker you may feel lightheaded due to your body's withdrawal from it; these symptoms will only last a few a days and will not be intense. If you have issues with your blood pressure be sure to consult your doctor.

3. Constipations

The best way to avoid this happening is by drinking lots of water and eating fiber rich vegetables; dark green vegetables are a good choice. You may also ingest a laxative if necessary.

4. Frequent urination

Initially you may notice that you are going to bathroom a bit more often, this is as a result of your body breaking down the excess glucose left in your body from previous carb intake. This sends a signal to the kidneys to push out excess water which results in you going to the bathroom more often. This will only last for a little while.

The side effects of the keto diet are quite minimal and may not be even affect everyone however it is good to be prepared in case you are affected. After all side effects on subsided your journey will progress smoothly and the benefits will certainly start to show.

Pros and Cons
I want to take all measures to make sure that the ketogenic experience is explained as thoroughly as possible to you as to avoid any hiccups going forward. Again this is not a quick fix diet and can even more so be view as a lifestyle change rather than dieting. As we go forward let us look into the pros and cons of this diet.

Pros

The keto diet can bring a host of benefits to the table, we will discuss a few.

17

1. **Blood sugar**

The LDL levels have been shown to decrease and these levels affect blood sugar. Diabetic individuals have reported recovering from their conditions.

2. **Energy**

You may see some increase in your energy levels as soon as you adapt to the keto diet. Fats are a great source of energy and since all meals are based on fat then your body will have more than enough resources to use up.

3. **Cholesterol**

Though you may eat more fats this has not shown to increase cholesterol levels but rather levels have been reported to be improved.

4. **Weight loss**

Of course with any diet the aim is to lose weight and the keto diet is no different. Though high in fats this does not affect weight loss. You will be able to see weight loss every single week that you are on the diet especially in the first month. Regaining weight will not be an issue as long as you stick to rational of eating high fat, low carb and moderate proteins.

Cons

The cons are really non-existent and are more so side effects that were discussed earlier in this chapter. As long as you are prepared for possible discomfort before your body can adapt then there really are no disadvantages to this diet.

Chapter 2

What to eat on the keto diet

With all this talk about high fat and low carbs what exactly will you be eating? What kind of fats and carbs are acceptable? This chapter will list some of the foods that you may have while on this diet.

Fats

Fats are the magic formula for the ketogenic follower and this does not mean oils. There are specific oils and fats that are acceptable for the diet. Some persons may not be able to ingest large amounts of mayonnaise or oil because it may affect them so those may be eliminated if those apply to you. Some foods contain Omega 6 fatty acids; try to avoid consuming these products as they promote inflammation within the body. Oils with Omega 6 should be heated and can be found in margarines, corn oil, nut oils, sunflower oil and canola oil. Not to worry there are many other options and these include:

- Mayonnaise (be sure to read label)
- Chicken fat (organic)
- Red palm oil
- Lard (organic)
- Butter (organic)
- Avocado oil
- Duck fat (organic)
- Olive oil
- Avocadoes
- Olives
- Ghee

❖   Coconut butter, cream and oil

Vegetables

Vegetables are the best way to cover your carb intake however
vegetables that are highly starchy should be avoided. Summer
squashes, potatoes, peas, corn and tomatoes should be avoided. Try to
choose from the following list:

❖   Celery
❖   Asparagus
❖   Cauliflower
❖   Bok Choy
❖   Green leafy veggies
❖   Sprouts
❖   Bamboo shoots
❖   Cabbage
❖   Kales
❖   Cucumbers
❖   Beetroot
❖   Mushrooms
❖   Shallots
❖   Turnips
❖   Collard greens
❖   Scallion
❖   Garlic
❖   Radishes
❖   Leeks
❖   Water chestnuts
❖   Chard
❖   Snow peas

Protein

You can get your protein from meats and seafood. Try not to choose lean meats but rather fatty cuts. You may choose from the list below.

- ❖ Eggs
- ❖ Soy products (be careful with soy products as they are high in carbs, be sure to measure precisely)
- ❖ Poultry : duck, quail, goose, Cornish hen, chicken, pheasant and turkey
- ❖ Pork
- ❖ Meat: veal, lamb, goat, beef and wild game.
- ❖ Protein powder with whey
- ❖ Sugar free bacon and sausage
- ❖ Fish and other seafood (avoid imitation crabmeat)

Dairy Products

Dairy products can also add protein component to your meals so be sure to use them in accordance with your daily requirements. Also it is best to choose dairy made with raw milk. You may choose from the list below:

- ❖ Cream cheese
- ❖ Full fat cottage cheese
- ❖ Mascarpone cheese
- ❖ Sour cream (full fat)
- ❖ Heavy whipping cream
- ❖ Hard and Soft Cheese (try to find cheeses that have 1 oz=1g carb)
- ❖ Yogurt (unsweetened, whole milk)

Seeds and Nuts

Nuts and seeds have oils within them which are a plus for the ketogenic follower; they are also great for snacking between meals. Peanuts are a no-no and other nuts should preferably be soaked and roasted before consumption. You can use flour that is made from nuts. The follow nuts are good choices:

- ❖ Walnuts
- ❖ Almonds
- ❖ Pecans
- ❖ Macadamia nuts
- ❖ Nut flours

Refreshments

It is important to keep hydrated while on the ketogenic diet as it helps to lessen the side effects. Water is the number one option but since the keto diet is not extremely restrictive some other liquids may be had, such as:

- ❖ Decaffeinated tea
- ❖ Unsweetened herbal tea
- ❖ Clear broth
- ❖ Decaf Coffee
- ❖ Limited amounts of lime/lemon juice
- ❖ Seltzer water (unsweetened, flavored)

Seasonings/spices

For flavor many of use various spices to season our foods, these seasonings also add to our carbs. There are some spices that even contain sugar. When using salt opt for sea salt as some regular brands contain dextrose.

- ❖ Cayenne pepper
- ❖ Cloves
- ❖ Mustard seeds
- ❖ Rosemary
- ❖ Black pepper
- ❖ Ground cinnamon
- ❖ Basil
- ❖ Dill
- ❖ Parsley
- ❖ Dry Cilantro/coriander seeds
- ❖ Ginger
- ❖ Turmeric
- ❖ Oregano
- ❖ Sage
- ❖ Chili pepper
- ❖ Thyme

Sweeteners

Though it is best to avoid all sugars and sweets, it is understandable that you may have a craving for something sweet sometimes. Avoid powdered sweeteners and opt for liquids instead. The following sweeteners are recommended:

- ❖ Monk fruit
- ❖ Erythritol
- ❖ Xylitol
- ❖ Splenda and Stevia liquid
- ❖ Inulin
- ❖ Chicory root

Well that was quite a list but I am sure you feel a bit at ease knowing exactly what to get to make your diet as simple as can be. Though this is quite an extensive list there may be some items that are not listed. With all the information that you have gathered I am sure that you will be able to spot other acceptable foods that you may consume.

Chapter 3

One Month Meal Plan

Meal Plan – Week One			
	Monday	**Tuesday**	**Wednesday**
Breakfast	Keto Oatmeal	Chicharrones con Huevos (Pork Rind and Eggs)	Keto Pancakes and Syrup
Lunch	Squash Spaghetti Lasagna Dish	Roasted Lemony Chicken & Prosciutto with Brussels sprouts	Slow Cooker Roast and Chicken Stew
Dinner	Smoky Pork Cassoulet	Seafood Stew	Curried Coconut Chicken Fingers
Thursday	**Friday**	**Saturday**	**Sunday**
Breakfast Berry Shake	Pizza Waffles	Red Pepper, Mozzarella and Bacon Frittata	Breakfast Quiche
Cheesy Zoodles with Fresh Basil	Oriental Garlicky Chicken Thighs	Pordenone Cauliflower Lasagna	Monterey Jack Steak
Cheeseburger Casserole	Curried Madras Lamb	Sage and Orange Glazed Duck	Chicken Parmesan

Meal Plan – Week Two			
	Monday	**Tuesday**	**Wednesday**
Breakfast	Cheesy Bacon and Chive Omelet	Bacon Avocado Breakfast Muffins	Orange Cinnamon Scones
Lunch	Keto Cheese Ocean Pizza	Baked Creamy Cauliflower-Broccoli Chicken	Pumpkin Chili
Dinner	Chicken Pot Pie	Beanless Chili con Carne	Baked Cheesy Meatballs
Thursday	**Friday**	**Saturday**	**Sunday**
Blueberry Almond Smoothie	Anaheim pepper Gruyere Waffles	Batter Coated Cheddar Cheese	Raspberry & Cacoa Breakfast Pudding
Spicy Spinach Casserole	Baked Manchego Chicken Wings	Bolognese Squash Spaghetti	Baked Pork Chops in Sweet-Sour Marinade
Slow Cooker Thai Fish Curry	Chicken & Endive Casserole	Herb Baked Salmon Fillets	Boneless Lamb Stew

Meal Plan – Week Three			
	Monday	**Tuesday**	**Wednesday**
Breakfast	Chicken Sausage and Pepper Jack Pie	Choco-Cashew Orange Smoothie	Keto Cheesy Boiled Eggs
Lunch	Chicken and Broccoli filled Zucchini	Chicken Angel Eggs	Super-Fast Egg Drop Soup
Dinner	Keto Butternut Squash Soup	Creamy Chicken Salad	Duck Breast with Balsamic Vinegar
Thursday	**Friday**	**Saturday**	**Sunday**
Mahón Kale Sausage Omelet Pie	Sour Cream Cheese Pancakes	Spicy Cauliflower with Sujuk Sausages	Strawberry Majoram Smoothie
Crispy Baked Tofu and Bok Choy Salad	Cheesy Bacon Spinach Log	Grilled Cheese and Ham Sandwich	Hearty Portobello Burgers
Stuffed Avocado with Tuna	Spinach Soup with Almonds and Parmesan	Lamb Cutlets with Garlic Sauce	Spiced Kale "Meatballs"

Meal Plan – Week Four			
	Monday	**Tuesday**	**Wednesday**
Breakfast	Vesuvius Scrambled Eggs with Provolone	Monterey Bacon-Scallions Omelet	Anaheim pepper Gruyere Waffles
Lunch	Bacon Chicken Patties	BBQ Chicken Soup	Beef Sausage, Bacon & Broccoli Casserole
Dinner	Zucchini Soup with Crunchy Cured Ham	Keto Paleo Almond Bread	Oriental Shrimp Soup
Thursday	**Friday**	**Saturday**	**Sunday**
Autumn Keto Pumpkin Bread	Smoked Turkey Bacon and Avocado Muffins	Anchovy, Spinach and Asparagus Omelet	Creamy Chocolate Milk
Homemade Meatballs	Salmon Salad in Avo Cups	Creamed Spinach	Cheesy Pizza
Spinach Soup with Almonds and Parmesan	Beef Cabbage Parsley Soup	Hot Mexican Meatballs	Seared Ribeye Steak

Chapter 4

I am sure you have been dying to see some of the recipes that you will be making. There are so many recipes that you can make on the keto diet. You will be pleasantly surprised at all the creative foods that will come of the kitchen once you begin preparing your meals. Feel free to double or triple or cut down on the serving of any recipe based on your liking. Remember it is fine to cook and freeze meals for eating later. I certainly hope you enjoy the recipes that are included below.

Happy cooking!!

Breakfast Recipes

Keto Pancakes and Syrup

Makes 10 (Serves 5)

Ingredients

For pancakes:

Eggs (4, large)

Erythritol (2 tablespoons)

Baking soda (1/2 teaspoon)

Nut butter of your choice (3/4 cup)

Coconut milk (1/3 cup)

Ghee (2 tablespoons)

Cinnamon powder (1 teaspoon)

For Syrup:

Maple extract (2 tablespoons, sugar-free)

Sukrin Fiber Syrup (1/2 cup)

Directions

1. Add ingredients for syrup to a jar and use spoon to stir until combined thoroughly. Cover jar and put aside until needed.
2. Put eggs, erythritol, baking soda, nut butter, coconut milk and cinnamon powder in a food processor and pulse until blended.
3. Heat ghee in a non-stick skillet and add batter to pot, use about ¼ cup per pancake. Cook until pancake sets then flip and finish cooking; place on a plate.
4. Repeat with remaining batter and plate.
5. Top with syrup and serve.

Nutritional Information

Calories 401

Net Carbs 3.6g

Fats 32.5g

Protein 12.8g

Fiber 5.3g

Cheesy Bacon and Chive Omelet

Makes 1

Ingredients

Bacon fat (1 teaspoon)

Cheddar cheese (1 oz.)

Salt

Bacon (2 slices, cooked)

Eggs (2, large)

Black pepper

Chives (2 stalks)

Directions

1. Beat eggs together and add pepper and salt to taste. Chop chives and shred cheese.
2. Heat skillet and cook bacon fat until hot.
3. Add eggs to pot and top with chives. Cook until edges start to set then add bacon and cook for 30-60 seconds.
4. Add cheese and use spatula to fold in half. Press to seal and flip over.
5. Warm and serve immediately.

Nutritional Information

Calories 463

Net Carbs 1g

Fats 39g

Protein 24g

Fiber 0g

Pizza Waffles

Makes 2

Ingredients

Parmesan cheese (4 tablespoons)

Psyllium husk powder (1 tablespoon)

Baking powder (1 teaspoon)

Salt

Cheddar cheese (3 oz.)

Eggs (4, large)

Almond flour (3 tablespoons)

Butter (1 tablespoon, organic)

Italian seasoning (1 teaspoon)-you may use a teaspoon of your preferred spices

Tomato sauce (1/2 cup)

Directions

1. Add all ingredients to a bowl except cheese and tomato sauce. Use mixer or immersion blender to combine until mixture is thick.

2. Heat waffle iron and use mixture to make two waffles.

3. Place waffles onto a lined baking sheet and top with tomato sauce and cheese (divide evenly). Broil for 3 minutes or until cheese melts.

4. Serve.

Nutritional Information

Calories 525.5

Net Carbs 5g

Fats 41.5g

Protein 29g

Fiber 5.5g

Breakfast Quiche

Ingredients

Coconut oil (3 tablespoons)

5 whole eggs

8 slices of bacon, cooked and chopped

100ml cream

Baby spinach, roughly chopped (2 cups)

Red pepper, chopped (1 cup)

Green pepper, chopped (1 cup)

Yellow onion, chopped (1 cup)

2 cloves of garlic, minced

Mushrooms, chopped (1 cup)

100g cheddar cheese, grated

salt to taste

Directions

1. Preheat oven at 375F

2. In a large bowl, mix all vegetables including the mushrooms together.

3. In another small bowl, whisk the 5 eggs with the cream

4. Carefully scoop the veggie mixture into a muffin pan coated with cooking spray, top with egg and cheese filling up to ¾ of the muffin tins. Sprinkle with chopped bacon on top.

5. Place in the oven to bake for 15 minutes or until the top of the quiche are firm.

6. Let it cook for a few minutes before serving.

Nutritional Information (1 small quiche)

Calories: 210

Net Carbs: 5g

Fat: 13g

Protein: 6g

Bacon Avocado Breakfast Muffins

Makes 16

Ingredients

Bacon (5 slices)

Almond flour (1/2 cup)

Psyllium husk powder (1 ½ tablespoons)

Colby Jack cheese (4.5 oz.)

Garlic (1 teaspoons, diced)

Chives (1 teaspoon, dried)

Salt

Lemon juice (1 ½ tablespoons)

Eggs (5)

Butter (2 tablespoons, organic)

Flaxseed meal (1/4 cup)

Avocados (2, cubed)

Spring onions (3)

Cilantro (1 teaspoon, dried)

Red chili flakes (1/4 teaspoon)

Coconut milk (1 ½ cup, from box)

Black Pepper

Baking powder (1 teaspoon)

Directions

1. Add flour, spices, lemon juice, eggs, flaxseed meal and coconut milk to a bowl. Mix together until thoroughly combined.
2. Heat a skillet and cook bacon until crispy then add the butter and avocado.
3. Add mixture to batter in bowl and mix together.
4. Set oven to 350 F and grease cupcake molds.
5. Add batter to molds and bake for 26 minutes. Take from oven and cool before removing from mold.
6. Serve. Store leftovers in fridge.

Nutritional Information

Calories 163

Net Carbs 1.5g

Fats 14.1g

Protein 6.1g

Fiber 3.3g

Chicharrones con Huevos (Pork Rind and Eggs)

Serves 3

Ingredients

Bacon (4 slices)

Pork Rinds (1.5 oz.)

Avocado (1, cubed)

Onion (1/4, chopped)

Salt

Eggs (5)

Tomato (1, chopped)

Jalapeno pepper (2, seeds removed and chopped)

Cilantro (1/4 cup, chopped)

Black pepper

Directions

1. Heat skillet and cook bacon until slightly crisp. Remove from pot and put aside on paper towels.
2. Add pork rinds to pot along with onion, tomatoes, pepper and cook for 3 minutes until onions are soft and clear.
3. Add cilantro, stir together gently and add eggs. Scramble eggs and then add avocado and fold.
4. Serve

Nutritional Information

Calories 508

Net Carbs 5g

Fats 43g

Protein 24.7g

Fiber 5.3g

Red Pepper, Mozzarella and Bacon Frittata

Serves 6

Ingredients

Olive oil (1 tablespoon)

Parsley (2 tablespoons, chopped)

Mozzarella cheese (4 oz., cubed)

Bell pepper (1, red, chopped)

Heavy cream (1/4 cup)

Salt

Bacon (7 slices)

Bella mushrooms (4 caps, large)

Basil (1/2 cup, chopped)

Goat cheese (2 oz., grated)

Eggs (9)

Parmesan cheese (1/4 cup, grated)

Black pepper

Directions

1. Set oven to 350 F.
2. Chop red pepper, bacon, basil and mushroom. Slice mozzarella into cubes and put aside.
3. Heat olive oil in a skillet until it slightly smokes then add bacon and cook for 5 minutes until browned.
4. Add red pepper and cook for 2 minutes until soft. While pepper cooks, add cream, parmesan cheese, eggs and black pepper to a bowl and whisk to combine.
5. Add mushrooms to pot, stir and cook for 5 minutes until soaked in fat. Add basil, cook for 1 minute then add mozzarella.
6. Put in egg mixture and use spoon to move ingredients around so that the egg gets on the bottom of pan.
7. Top with goat cheese and place in oven for 8 minutes then broil for 6 minutes.
8. Use knife to pry frittata edges from pan and place on a plate and slice.
9. Serve.

Nutritional Information

Calories 408

Net Carbs 2.4g

Fats 31.2g

Protein 19.2g

Fiber 0.8g

Cheese and Sausage Pies

Serves 2

Ingredients

Cheddar cheese (3/4 cup, grated)

Coconut oil (1/4 cup)

Egg yolks (5)

Rosemary (1/2 teaspoon)

Baking soda (1/4 teaspoon)

Chicken sausage (1 ½)

Coconut flour (1/4 cup)

Coconut milk (2 tablespoons)

Lemon juice (2 teaspoons)

Cayenne pepper (1/4 teaspoon)

Kosher salt (1/8 teaspoon)

Directions

1. Set oven to 350 F.
2. Chop sausage, heat skillet and cook sausage. While sausages cook combine all dry ingredients in a bowl. In another bowl combine lemon juice, oil and coconut milk. Add liquids to dry mixture and add ½ cup of cheese; fold to combine and put into 2 ramekins.
3. Add cooked sausages to batter and use spoon to push into mixture.
4. Bake for 25 minutes until golden on top. Top with leftover cheese and broil for 4 minutes.
5. Serve warm.

Nutritional Information

Calories 711

Net Carbs 5.8g

Fats 65.3g

Protein 34.3g

Fiber 11.5g

Keto Oatmeal

Serves 2

Ingredients

Chia seeds (1/4 cup)

Coconut flakes (1/3 cup, unsweetened)

Vanilla (1 teaspoon, sugar free)

Almond milk (1 cup, unsweetened)

Stevia extract (10 drops)

Coconut (1/4 cup, shredded, unsweetened)

Almonds (1/3 cup, flaked)

Heavy whipping cream (1/2 cup)

Erythritol (2 tablespoons)

Directions

1. Place almond and coconut flakes in a pot and toast for 3 minutes until fragrant.
2. Place toasted ingredients into a bowl along with chia seeds, erythritol and shredded coconut; mix together to combine.
3. Top with milk and stir. You can use hot or cold milk based on your preference.
4. Add vanilla and stevia, stir and set aside for 5-10 minutes.
5. Serve. May be topped with fresh berries.

Nutritional Information

Calories 359

Net Carbs 5g

Fats 30.4g

Protein 9.4 g

Fiber 10.5g

Breakfast Berry Shake

Serves 3

Ingredients

Mixed berries (3/4 cup)

Almond milk (1 cup)

All-natural peanut butter (1 tablespoon)

Protein powder (1 tablespoon)

Cinnamon powder (1/4 teaspoons)

Ginger, minced (1/4 teaspoons)

Directions

1. Place all the ingredients in a blender and mix until smooth.

Nutritional Information

Calories: 319

Net Carbs: 9g

Fat: 15g

Protein: 28g

Breakfast Tacos

Serves 3

Ingredients

Eggs (6)

Bacon (3 strips)

Cheddar cheese (1 oz., shredded)

Mozzarella cheese (1 cup, shredded)

Butter (2 tablespoons)

Avocado (1/2, cubed)

Salt

Black pepper

Directions

1. Cook bacon until crisp, put aside until needed.
2. Heat a non-stick pan and place 1/3 cup mozzarella into pan and cook for 3 minutes until browned around the edges. Place a wooden spoon across a bowl or pot and use tongs to lift cheese 'taco from pot. Repeat with leftover cheese.
3. Melt butter in a skillet and scramble eggs; use pepper and salt to season.
4. Spoon eggs into hardened shells and top with avocado and bacon.
5. Top with cheddar and serve.

Nutritional Information

Calories 443

Net Carbs 3g

Fats 36.2g

Protein 25.7 g

Fiber 1.7g

Raspberry & Cacoa Breakfast Pudding

Serves 1

Ingredients

Cacao powder (1 tablespoon)

Raspberry (1/4 cups)

Chia seeds (3 tablespoon)

Almond milk (1 cup)

Agave or Xylitol (1 teaspoon)

Directions

1. In a small bowl, combine the almond milk and cacao powder. Stir well.

2. Add the chia seeds to the bowl and let it rest for 5 minutes.

3. Using a fork, fluff the chia and cacao mixture and then place in the fridge to chill for at least 30 minutes.

4. Serve with raspberries and a drizzle of agave on top

Nutritional Information

Calories 230

Net Carbs 4g

Fats 20g

Protein 15 g

Orange Cinnamon Scones

Serves 8

Ingredients
For Scones:

Heavy cream (1/3 cup)

Butter (1/4 cup, unsalted, cubed)

Coconut oil (2 tablespoons)

Golden Flaxseed (1 tablespoon)

Cinnamon (1 ½ teaspoons)

Xanthan (1/4 teaspoon)

Salt (1/4 teaspoon)

Coconut flour (8 tablespoons)

Erythitol (1/4 cup)

Eggs (2)

Maple syrup (2 tablespoons)-recipe above

Baking powder (1 ½ teaspoons)

Vanilla (1 teaspoon)

Stevia (1/4 teaspoon)

Orange zest (from 1 orange)

For Icing:

Stevia (20 drops)

Orange juice (1 tablespoon)

Coconut butter (1/4 cup)

Directions

1. Set oven to 400 °F.
2. Place all dry ingredients in a bowl except xanthan and 1 tablespoon flour. Add butter and oil to dry mix and stir to combine.
3. Combine sweetener and eggs until thoroughly mixed and light in color. Put in maple syrup, remaining flour, xanthan gum, heavy cream and vanilla; mix until combined and thick.
4. Add wet mixture to dry, reserving 2 tablespoons of liquids, mix together and add cinnamon and use hands to form mixture into dough. Shape into a ball and press into a cake like shape. Slice into 8 pieces.
5. Place onto a lined baking sheet and use reserved liquid to brush the top of scones.
6. Bake for 15 minutes, remove from oven and cool.
7. Prepare icing and drizzle over scones before serving.

Nutritional Information

Calories 232

Net Carbs 3.3g

Fats 20g

Protein 3.3 g

Fiber 4.3g

Blueberry Almond Smoothie

Serves 2

Ingredients

Unsweetened almond milk (16 ounces)

Xylitol (1 teaspoon)

Heavy cream (4 ounces)

Frozen unsweetened blueberries (1/4 cup)

Whey Vanilla protein powder (1 scoop)

Directions

1. Put all ingredients in blender and blend until smooth.
2. Add a little water if it becomes too thick.
3. Measure those blueberries as they add more carbs.

Nutritional Information

Calories 302

Net Carbs 6g

Fats 25g

Protein 15g

Fiber 1g

Creamy Chocolate Milk

Serves 2

Ingredients

Unsweetened almond milk (16 ounces)

Xylitol (1 teaspoon)

Heavy cream (4 ounces)

Whey Chocolate Isolate powder (1 scoop)

Crushed ice (1/2 cup) (optional: add if you like a thick drink, but the flavor will be less intense.)

Directions

1. Put all ingredients in blender and blend until smooth.
2. This recipe can be doubled, as can most low carb smoothie recipes.

Nutritional Information

Calories 292

Net Carbs 4g

Fats 25g

Protein 15 g

Anaheim pepper Gruyere Waffles

Serves: 2

Ingredients

1 small Anheim pepper

3 eggs

1/4 cup cream cheese

1/4 cup Gruyere cheese

1 Tbsp coconut flour

1 tsp Metamucil powder

1 tsp baking powder

salt and pepper to tast

Directions

1. In a blender, mix together all ingredients except for the cheese and anaheim pepper. Once the ingredients are mixed well, add cheese and pepper. Blend well until all ingredients are unit well.
2. Heat your waffle iron; pour on the waffle mix and cook 5-6 minutes. Serve hot.

Nutritional Information

Calories 223.55

Net Carbs 5.50g

Fats 17g

Protein 11 g

Anchovy, Spinach and Asparagus Omelet

Serves: 2

Ingredients

2 organic eggs

3/4 cup of spinach

2 oz anchovy in olive oil

4 marinated asparagus

Celtic Sea salt

Freshly ground black pepper

Directions

1. Preheat the oven to 375 F.
2. In the bottom of the baking pan place the anchovy.
3. In a bowl, beat the eggs and pou on top of the fish. Add the spinach and the chopped asparagus on top.
4. Season with salt and pepper to taste.
5. Bake in preheated oven for about 10 minutes.
6. Serve hot.

Cooking Times

Total Time: 15 minutes

Nutritional Information

Calories 83

Net Carbs 2.28g

Fats 4.91g

Protein 7.5 g

Autumn Keto Pumpkin Bread

Serves: 8

Ingredients

3 egg whites

1/2 cup coconut milk

1 1/2 cup almond flour

1/2 cup pumpkin puree

2 tsp baking powder

1 1/2 tsp Pumpkin pie spice

1/2 tsp Kosher Salt

coconut oil for greasing

Directions

1. Preheat your oven to 350F. Grease a standard bread loaf pan with melted coconut oil.
2. Sift all dry ingredients into a large bowl.
3. In another bowl, add pumpkin puree and coconut milk and mix well. In a separate bowl, beat the egg whites. Fold in egg whites and gently fold into the dough.
4. Spread the dough into the prepared bread pan.
5. Bake the bread for 75 minutes. Once ready, remove bread from the oven and let cool.
6. Slice and serve.

Cooking Times

Total Time: 1 hour and 25 minutes

Nutritional Information

Calories 197

Net Carbs 8.18g

Fats 16g

Protein 7.2 g

Batter Coated Cheddar Cheese

Serves: 1

Ingredients

1 large egg

2 slices Cheddar cheese (3.55 oz)

1 tsp ground walnuts

1 tsp ground flaxseed

2 tsp almond flour

1 tsp hemp seeds

1 Tbsp olive oil

Salt and pepper to taste

Directions

1. In a small bowl, whisk an egg together with the salt and pepper.
2. Heat a tablespoon of olive oil in a frying pan, on medium heat.
3. In a separate bowl, mix the ground flaxseed with the ground walnuts, hemp seeds and the almond flour.
4. Coat the cheddar slices with the egg mix, then roll in the dry mix and fry cheese for about 3 minutes on each side. Serve hot.

Cooking Times

Total Time: 13 minutes

Nutritional Information

Calories 509

Net Carbs 2g

Fats 16g

Protein 21 g

Chicken Sausage and Pepper Jack Pie

Serves: 5

Ingredients

5 egg yolks

1 1/2 chicken sausage

3/4 cup Pepper Jack cheese

1/4 cup coconut flour

2 tsp lime Juice

1/2 tsp dried basil

1/4 tsp baking soda

4 Tbs coconut oil

2 Tbsp coconut water

Kosher salt to taste

Directions

1. Preheat oven to 350F.
2. In a frying pan add the sausages and cook on medium high heat 3-4 minutes. Set aside.
3. Measure out the dry ingredients into a bowl.
4. Separate 5 egg yolks from the whites, then discard of the whites.
5. Beat the egg yolks about 4-5 minutes. Add in coconut oil, coconut water, and lime juice. Continue to beat again until smooth and creamy.

6. Mix the wet ingredients into the dry ingredients slowly. At last, add cheese into the batter.
7. Measure out the batter into 2 ramekins. Poke the sausages into the batter.
8. Bake in preheated oven for 25 minutes. Once ready, serve hot.

Cooking Times

Total Time: 40 minutes

Nutritional Information

Calories 294

Net Carbs 7.66g

Fats 24g

Protein 11 g

Choco-Cashew Orange Smoothie

Serves: 1

Ingredients

1 cup cashew milk

1 handful of arugula leaves

1 Tbsp chocolate whey protein powder

1/8 tsp orange extract

Ice cubes

Directions

1. Place all ingredients in your blender and blend until well united and smooth.
2. Add extra ice and serve.

Cooking Times

Total Time: 5 minutes

Nutritional Information

Calories 45

Net Carbs 7g

Fats 1.05g

Protein 3 g

Coffee Ketocino

Serves: 1

Ingredients

1 cup cold coffee

1/3 cup heavy cream

1/4 tsp xantham gum

1 tsp pure vanilla extract

2 Tbsp Xylitol

6 ice cubes

Directions

1. Place all ingredients in your blender.
2. Blend until all unite well and become smooth.
3. Serve.

Cooking Times

Total Time: 5 minutes

Nutritional Information

Calories 287

Net Carbs 2.76g

Fats 29g

Protein 1.91 g

Keto Cheesy Boiled Eggs

Serves: 2

Ingredients

3 eggs

2 Tbsp almond butter, no-stir

2 Tbsp softened cream cheese

1 tsp whipping cream

Salt and pepper to taste

Directions

1. In a small saucepan hard boil the eggs.
2. When ready, wash the eggs with cold wate, peel and chop them. Place eggs in a bowl; add in the butter, cream cheese and whipping cream.
3. Mix well and add salt and pepper to taste. Serve.

Cooking Times

Total Time: 20 minutes

Nutritional Information

Calories 212

Net Carbs 0.75g

Fats 19g

Protein 7 g

Mahón Kale Sausage Omelet Pie

Serves: 8

Ingredients

10 eggs

1 1/2 cup Mahón cheese (or Cheddar)

3 chicken sausages

3 cups raw chopped Kale leaves

2 1/2 cup mushrooms, chopped

1 Tbsp garlic powder

2 tsp Hot sauce

1/2 tsp black pepper and celery seed

salt and pepper to taste

Directions

1. Preheat oven to 400F.
2. Chop up your sausage and mushroom thin and place them in a cast iron skillet. Cook on a medium-high heat for 2-3 minutes.
3. While the sausages are cooking, chop your spinach up. Add in a skillet the mushrooms and spinach.
4. In a meanwhile, in a bowl mix eggs with black pepper and celery seed, hot sauce, and spices. Scramble them well.
5. Mix your sausages, spinach, and mushrooms so that the spinach can wilt fully. Add salt and pepper to taste.
6. Finally, add the cheese to the top.
7. Pour your eggs over the mixture and mix everything well.

8. Stir the mixture for a few seconds, and then put your cast iron skillet in the oven. Bake for 10-12 minutes, and then broil the top for 3-4 minutes.
9. Let cool for a while, cut into 8 slices and serve hot.

Cooking Times

Total Time: 25 minutes

Nutritional Information

Calories 266

Net Carbs 7g

Fats 17g

Protein 19 g

Monterey Bacon-Scallions Omelet

Serves: 2

Ingredients

2 eggs

2 slices cooked bacon

1/4 cup scallions, chopped

1/4 cup Monterey jack cheese

salt and pepper to taste

1 tsp lard

Directions

1. In a frying pan heat lard in on medium-low heat. Add the eggs, scallions and salt and pepper to taste.
2. Cook for 1-2 minutes; add the bacon and sauté 30 - 45 seconds longer. Turn the heat off on the stove.
3. On top of the bacon place a cheese. Then, take two edges of the omelet and fold them onto the cheese. Hold the edges there for a moment as the cheese has to partially melt. Make the same with the other egg and let cook in a warm pan for a while.
4. Serve hot.

Cooking Times

Total Time: 15 minutes

Nutritional Information

Calories 321

Net Carbs 1.62g

Fats 28g

Protein 14 g

Smoked Turkey Bacon and Avocado Muffins

Serves: 16

Ingredients

5 eggs

6 slices smoked turkey bacon

1/2 cup almond flour

2 medium Avocados

1/2 cup Cheddar cheese

1 1/2 cup coconut milk

3 spring onions

1 tsp minced garlic

2 tsp dried parsley

1/4 tsp red chili powder

1 1/2 Tbsp lemon juice

1/4 cup flaxseed

1 1/2 Tbsp Metamucil powder

1 tsp baking powder

2 Tbsp butter

salt and pepper to taste

Directions

1. Preheat oven to 350F.
2. In a frying pan over medium-low heat, cook the bacon with the butter until crisp. Add the spring onions, cheese, and baking powder.
3. In a bowl, mix together coconut milk, eggs, Metamucil powder, almond flour, flax, spices and lemon juice. Switch off the heat and let cool. Then, crumble the bacon and add all of the fat to the egg mixture.
4. Clean and chop avocado and fold into the mixture.
5. Measure out batter into a cupcake tray that's been sprayed or greased with nonstick spray and bake for 25-26 minutes.
6. Once ready, let cool and serve hot or cold.

Cooking Times

Total Time: 40 minutes

Nutritional Information

Calories 184

Net Carbs 5.51g

Fats 16g

Protein 5.89 g

Sour Cream Cheese Pancakes

Serves: 2

Ingredients

2 eggs

1/4 cup cream cheese

1 Tbsp coconut flour

1 tsp ground ginger

1/2 cup liquid Stevia

coconut oil

sugar-free maple syrup

Directions

1. In a deep bowl, beat together all of the ingredients until smooth.
2. Heat up a frying skillet with oil on medium-high. Ladle the batter and pour in hot oil.
3. Cook on one side and then flip. Top with a sugar-free maple syrup and serve.

Cooking Times

Total Time: 15 minutes

Nutritional Information

Calories 170

Net Carbs 4g

Fats 13g

Protein 6.90 g

Spicy Cauliflower with Sujuk Sausages

Serves: 4

Ingredients

4 cups frozen cauliflower

8 oz sujuk sausages sliced (or red pastrami)

1 green pepper, chopped

1 tsp cajun seasoning

1/2 onion, chopped

2 Tbsp minced garlic

2 Tbsp olive oil

Directions

1. In a frying pan, sauté onion with olive oil for 2-3 minutes.
2. Squeeze the liquid from chopped cauliflower and add it to the pan. Sauté the cauliflower with onion 5-10 minutes.
3. Add in cajun seasoning and mix. Add in chopped sujuk sausages or pastrami and green peppers.
4. Toss and cook until about 5 minutes. Transfer to the plates. Serve.

Cooking Times

Total Time: 20 minutes

Nutritional Information

Calories 181

Net Carbs 9g

Fats 10g

Protein 14 g

Strawberry Majoram Smoothie

Serves: 1

Ingredients

1/4 cup fresh or frozen strawberries

2 fresh marjoram leaf

2 Tbs heavy cream

1 cup unsweetened coconut milk

1 Tbs sugar-free vanilla syrup

1/2 tsp pure vanilla extract

ice cubes (optional)

Directions

1. Place all ingredients in your blender and mix until become smooth.
2. If you wish you can add the ice cubes. Serve.

Cooking Times

Total Time: 5 minutes

Nutritional Information

Calories 292

Net Carbs 6g

Fats 26.7g

Protein 2.8 g

Fiber 0.76g

Vesuvius Scrambled Eggs with Provolone

Serves: 2

Ingredients

2 large eggs

3/4 cup Provolone cheese

1.76 oz air-dried salami

1 tsp fresh rosemary (chopped)

1 Tbsp Olive oil

Salt and pepper to taste

Directions

1. In a small pan with olive oil fry the chopped salami.
2. In the meantime, in a small bowl whisk the eggs, then add the salt, pepper and fresh rosemary.
3. Add in the provolone cheese and mix well with a fork.
4. Pour the egg mixture to the pan with salami and cook for about 5 minutes. Serve hot.

Cooking Times

Total Time: 10 minutes

Nutritional Information

Calories 374

Net Carbs 2.4g

Fats 30g

Protein 22.4 g

Fiber 0.27g

Lunch Recipes

Tuna Avocado Bites

Makes 12

Ingredients

Mayonnaise (1/4 cup)

Parmesan cheese (1/4 cup)

Garlic powder (1/2 teaspoon)

Salt

Canned Tuna (10 oz., drained)

Avocado (1, cubed)

Almond flour (1/3 cup)

Onion powder (1/4 teaspoon)

Coconut oil (1/2 cup)

Directions

1. Combine all ingredients in a bowl except oil and avocado.
2. Add avocado and fold, use hands to form balls and dust with flour.
3. Heat oil in a pot and fry tuna bites until golden all over.
4. Serve.

Nutritional Information per bite

Calories 135

Net Carbs 0.8g

Fats 11.8g

Protein 6.2 g

Fiber 1.2g

N.B- 3-4 bites would be good for a serving. Paired with a salad and lunch is complete.

Crispy Baked Tofu and Bok Choy Salad

Serves 3

Ingredients

For Tofu:

Soy sauce (1 tablespoon)

Water (1 tablespoon)

Rice wine vinegar (1 tablespoon)

Tofu (15 oz., extra firm)

Sesame oil (1 tablespoon)

Garlic (2 teaspoons)

Lemon juice (from ½ lemon)

For Salad:

Green onion (1 stalk)

Coconut oil (3 tablespoons)

Sambal Olek (1 tablespoon)

Lime juice (from ½ lime)

Bok Choy (9 oz.)

Cilantro (2 tablespoons, chopped)

Soy sauce (2 tablespoons)

Peanut butter (1 tablespoon)

Stevia liquid (7 drops)

Directions

1. Wrap tofu in a clean cloth and press for 6 hours until dry.
2. Combine soy sauce, water, vinegar, lemon juice, sesame oil and garlic in a bowl and cube tofu. Add to marinade, cover with plastic and put aside for 30 minutes or overnight if possible.
3. Set oven to 350 F. Use parchment paper to line a baking sheet and place marinated tofu on sheet. Bake for 35 minutes.
4. Prepare dressing for salad by combining all ingredients except bok choy. Chop bok choy finely and toss in dressing.
5. Top bok choy with baked tofu and serve.

Nutritional Information

Calories 442

Net Carbs 5.7g

Fats 35g

Protein 25 g

Fiber 1.7g

Homemade Meatballs

Serves 6

Ingredients

500g ground beef

1 whole egg

Almond flour (1/2 cups)

2 cloves of garlic, minced

Oregano, dried (1 teaspoon)

Thyme, dried (1 teaspoon)

1 cup mozzarella cheese, shredded

Salt and pepper to taste

Homemade marinara sauce (1/2 cups)

Directions

1. Preheat oven at 450F.

2. In a large bowl, place the ground beef, egg, almond flour, garlic, oregano, thyme, and season with salt and pepper. Also add the cheese.

3. Using your hands, mix all the ingredients together, making sure that everything is well combined.

4. Create 25 pcs of meat balls and lay them on a baking sheet lined with parchment paper.

5. Cook in the oven to cook for 15 minutes or until golden brown.

6. Serve the meatballs with marinara sauce.

Nutritional Information

Calories: 117

Net Carbs: 0.9

Fat: 9.3g

Protein: 7g

BBQ Chicken Soup

Serves 4

Ingredients

For Soup Base:

Chicken thighs (3)

Salt

Chicken broth (1 ½ cups)

Chili seasoning (2 teaspoons)

Olive oil (2 tablespoons)

Beef broth (1 ½ cups)

Black pepper

For BBQ Sauce:

Ketchup (1/4 cup, reduced sugar)

Dijon mustard (2 tablespoons)

Hot sauce (1 tablespoon)

Worcestershire sauce (1 teaspoon)

Onion powder (1 teaspoon)

Red chili flakes (1 teaspoon)

Butter (1/4 cup)

Tomato paste (1/4 cup)

Soy sauce (1 tablespoon)

Liquid smoke (2 ½ teaspoons)

Garlic powder (1 ½ teaspoons)

Chili powder (1 teaspoon)

Cumin (1 teaspoon)

Directions

1. Set oven to 400 F. Remove bones from chicken and put bones aside. Season chicken with chili seasoning and place into oven for 50 minutes.
2. Heat oil in a deep pot and add bones. Cook for 5 minutes then add beef and chicken broth; season with pepper and salt.
3. Take chicken from oven and remove skin. Add the fat to the soup and mix together. Combine BBQ sauce ingredients and add to pot. Cook for 30 minutes.
4. Combine fats in soup by using an immersion blender then shred chicken and add to soup. Cook for 20 minutes.
5. Serve topped with chicken skin. May add cheese or bell peppers.

Nutritional Information

Calories 487

Net Carbs 4.3g

Fats 38.3g

Protein 24.5 g

Fiber 1.3g

Salmon Salad in Avo Cups

Serves 2

Ingredients

1 medium-sized salmon fillet

1 pc. shallot, diced

Mayo (1/4 cups)

½ juice of lime

Fresh dill, chopped (2 tablespoons)

Ghee (1 tablespoon)

1 large avocado, sliced in half and pitted

salt and pepper to taste

Directions

1. Preheat oven at 400F

2. Place the salmon fillet on a baking sheet and drizzle it with ghee and juice of lime. Season with salt and pepper and place in the oven to cook for 20-25 minutes.

3. When done, allow the salmon to cook for a few minutes and shred using a fork.

4. Place the salmon in a bowl, add the diced shallot, and mix well.

5. Add the dill and mayo to the salmon mixture and combine well. Set aside.

6.   Remove the insides of the avocado halves making sure that the skin is still intact to make cups.

7.   Mash the avocado meat in a bowl and then add to the salmon mixture. Combine well.

8.   Transfer the avocado and salmon salad back to the avocado cups and serve.

Nutritional Information

Calories: 463

Net Carbs: 6.4g

Fat: 35g

Protein: 27g

Bacon Chicken Patties

Serves 10

Ingredients

Chicken breast (12 oz. can)

Bell peppers (2, medium)

Parmesan cheese (1/4 cup)

Coconut flour (3 tablespoons)

Bacon (4 slices)

Sundried Tomato pesto (1/4 cup)

Egg (1)

Directions

1. Cook bacon until crisp, put aside until needed.
2. Put bell pepper into a processor and pulse until fine, put into a bowl and squeeze out excess liquid.
3. Put bacon and chicken into processor and pulse until thoroughly combined, transfer mixture to bowl with peppers.
4. Add egg, pesto parmesan and flour to mixture and combine.
5. Heat oil in a skillet and form patties. Add to pan and cook until golden all over.
6. Serve.

Nutritional Information per patty

Calories 159

Net Carbs 1.7g

Fats 11.5g

Protein 9.9 g

Fiber 14g

Savoury Mince

Serves 5

Ingredients

Coconut oil (4 tablespoons)

1Kg Beef/Chicken/Lamb/Pork/Ostrich mince

2 Onion finely diced

Vegetables (green/red/yellow/orange peppers, mushroom, tomatoes, celery, baby marrows, spinach) finely diced (4 cups)

4 Carrots finely grated

1 Packet gluten free gravy

Tomato paste (1/2 cups)

250ml chicken stock

Directions

1. Heat coconut oil in a pan and fry chopped onion,

2. Add beef mince with and tomato paste and fry.

3. Add chopped vegetables and grated carrot to the cooked mince.

4. Continue to cook on a low heat until the vegetables are well cooked.

5. If your mixture seems to be drying out, keep adding chicken stock to keep at the right consistency.

6. The longer you cook this mixture, the more the flavors will infuse through the mince.

7. Add gluten free gravy.

Cheesy Bacon Spinach Log

Serves 5

Ingredients

Cheddar cheese (2 ½ cups, shredded)

Chipotle seasoning (2 tablespoons)

Bacon (30 slices)

Mrs. Dash seasoning (2 teaspoons)

Spinach (5 cups)

Directions

1. Set oven to 375 °F.
2. Place bacon in a weaving pattern on a baking sheet lined with foil and season with spices.
3. Top bacon with cheese leaving a 1 inch space all around the edge. Add spinach and push it down and roll the bacon together into a log.
4. Sprinkle with salt and place into oven for 60 minutes.
5. Cool for 15 minutes and slice.
6. Serve.

Nutritional Information

Calories 432

Net Carbs 3g

Fats 38.2g

Protein 32.8 g

Fiber 3g

Beef Sausage, Bacon & Broccoli Casserole

Ingredients

500 g beef sausage

1/2 head of broccoli

8 slices of bacon

Cream (1/2 cups)

Dijon mustard (1 tablespoon)

100 g grated cheddar cheese

Directions

1. Preheat oven to 350F

2. Slice the sausage and place in a small baking dish.

3. Slice the bacon and add to the sausage.

4. Break the broccoli into florets and arrange between the meat.

5. Mix the cream and mustard in a bowl and pour it all over the casserole, then top with the cheese.

6. Bake in the oven for 35 minutes.

Nutritional Information

Calories: 300

Net Carbs: 3g

Fat: 25g

Protein: 20g

Grilled Cheese and Ham Sandwich

Ingredients

For buns:

Eggs (2)

Salted butter (1 ½ tablespoons)

Coconut flour (1 teaspoon)

Almond flour (3/4 cup)

Coconut oil (2 tablespoons)

Baking powder (1 teaspoon)

Salt (1/4 teaspoon)

Filling:

Deli Ham (4 slices)

Cheddar cheese (2 slices)

Butter (1 tablespoon, salted)

Muenster cheese (2 slices)

Directions

1. Set oven to 350 F.
2. Place almond flour, baking powder in a bowl and mix together.

3. Put coconut oil and butter in a microwavable dish and heat until melted then add to dry mix. Combine until mixture gets doughy.
4. Beat eggs and add to dough mixture then put in coconut flour.
5. Grease cupcake molds and add batter to each about ¾ ways filled. Baked for 18 minutes and take from oven, allow to cool and slice into two horizontally.
6. Use cheese and ham to fill buns, melt butter in a skillet and place sandwiches into pan. Cook for 3 minutes on each side until golden and cheese melts.
7. Serve.

Nutritional Information

Calories 272

Net Carbs 1.8g

Fats 24.2g

Protein 11.3g

Fiber 3.8g

Creamed Spinach

Serves 1

Ingredients

Spinach (2 cups)

½ small onion, chopped

Water (1/4 cups)

1/2 stock cube

1 clove of garlic, chopped

Heavy cream (1/4 cups)

Butter (2 tablespoons)

Salt and pepper to taste

Directions

1. Place spinach and onion to a pan with water and heat over medium-high fire.

2. Add stock cube and garlic and allow to steam for 8-10 minutes or until all the water has evaporated and the spinach is very soft.

3. Pour in the heavy cream and butter and then season with salt and pepper. Cooking until it thickens.

4. Using a hand-held blender blitz the spinach until fairly smooth.

5. Serve while hot

Nutritional Information

Calories: 200

Net Carbs: 3g

Fat: 23g

Protein: 7g

Cheesy Pizza

Makes 12 small slices

Ingredients

Ground beef (1/2 lb.)

Eggs (2)

Garlic powder (1 teaspoon)

Basil (1/4 teaspoon)

Turmeric (1/4 teaspoon)

Cream cheese (8 oz., room temp.)

Chorizo sausage (1)

Parmesan cheese (1/4 cup, grated)

Cumin (1/2 teaspoon)

Italian seasoning (1/2 teaspoon)

Tomato sauce (3/4 cup, low carb)

Salt

Black pepper

Directions

1. Set oven to 375°F.
2. Put cream cheese, eggs, garlic powder, parmesan cheese and black pepper in a bowl and use mixer to blend until smooth.
3. Grease a baking pan and pour in cheese mixture and spread evenly; bake for 15 minutes.
4. Put beef into a skillet and cook for 5 minutes then add Italian seasoning, basil, salt, black pepper, cumin and turmeric. Cook for 10 minutes or until thoroughly cooked.
5. Take crust from oven and cool for 10 minutes then top with tomato sauce and cheese. Return to oven and bake for 10 minutes until cheese melts then top with beef.
6. Broil for an additional 5 minutes. Take from oven and cool for 10 minutes.
7. Slice and serve.

Nutritional Information per slice

Calories 145

Net Carbs 1.2g

Fats 11.3g

Protein 8.2 g

Fiber 3g

Hearty Portobello Burgers

Serves 1

Ingredients

Coconut oil (1/2 tablespoon)

Oregano (1 teaspoon)

Portobello mushroom caps (2)

Garlic (1 clove)

Salt

Black pepper

Dijon mustard (1 tablespoon)

Cheddar cheese (1/4 cup)

Beef/bison (6 oz.)

Directions

1. Heat griddle and combine spices and oil in a bowl.
2. Remove gills from mushrooms and place into marinade until needed.
3. Add beef, cheese, salt, mustard and pepper in another bowl and mix to combine; form into a patty.
4. Place marinated caps onto grill and cook for 8 minutes until thoroughly heated. Place patty onto grill and cook on each side for 5 minutes.
5. Take 'buns' from grill and top with burger and any other toppings you choose.

6. Serve.

Nutritional Information

Calories 735

Net Carbs 4g

Fats 48g

Protein 60g

Fiber 4g

Chicken and Broccoli filled Zucchini

Serves 2

Ingredients

Butter (2 tablespoons)

Broccoli (1 cup)

Sour cream (2 tablespoons)

Zucchini (10 oz.)-2

Cheddar cheese (3 oz., shredded)

Rotisserie chicken (6 oz., shredded)

Green onion (1 stalk)

Salt

Black pepper

Directions

1. Set oven to 400 F.
2. Slice zucchinis in half lengthwise and use spoons to remove cores. Melt butter and pour equally into each zucchini shell. Add black pepper and salt and bake for 20 minutes.
3. Chop broccoli and place into a bowl with sour cream and chicken. Fill zucchini boats with chicken mixture and top with cheese.
4. Bake for 15 minutes more or until golden.
5. Serve topped with green onion.

Nutritional Information

Calories 476.5

Net Carbs 5g

Fats 34g

Protein 30 g

Fiber 3g

Super-Fast Egg Drop Soup

Serves 1

Ingredients

Chicken broth (1 ½ cups)

Butter (1 tablespoon)

Chili garlic paste (1 teaspoon)

Chicken bouillon (1/2 cube)

Eggs (2)

Directions

1. Add butter to pan, heat until it melts then add broth and bouillon
2. Bring to a boil and add chili paste, stir to combine and remove from flame.
3. Beat eggs in a bowl and add to broth, stir and put aside for a few minutes.
4. Serve.

Nutritional Information

Calories 279

Net Carbs 2.5g

Fats 23g

Protein 12g

Baked Creamy Cauliflower-Broccoli Chicken

Serves: 8

Ingredients

2 boneless chicken breasts

1 cup chicken broth

3 cups cauliflower

3 cups broccoli, steamed and chopped

2 cups shredded Cheddar cheese

1 cup heavy cream

1 small yellow onion

1/2 Tbsp minced garlic

1 tsp lemon juice

1/2 cup mayonnaise

3 Tbsp ghee

fresh parsley, chopped

salt and fresh pepper to taste

Directions

1. Preheat the oven to 350 degrees.
2. In a deep saucepot boil chicken breast until the chicken is cooked through.
3. Meanwhile, in a frying pan with the ghee cook up the garlic and onions on a low heat. Add all spices one by one stirring frequently.
4. While that's cooking, in a food processor blend up your cauliflower.
5. When the onions are soft, add the cauliflower. Cook for 2-3 minutes. Add in the chicken broth. Cook, covered for about 10 minutes.
6. Add the heavy cream and lemon juice and let simmer uncovered on low for about 10 minutes more. At the end, add in mayonnaise and stir.
7. Pull apart your chicken and add half of chicken into the cauliflower cream mixture.
8. Use the other half to line the bottom of an 8x8 casserole dish.On top of the chicken, layer in chopped broccoli.
9. Top with the cauliflower cream mixture.
10. Cover it with cheddar cheese.
11. Bake in preheated oven for 40 minutes. Serve hot.

Cooking Times

Total Time: 1 hour and 15 minutes

Nutritional Information

Calories 365

Net Carbs 9.2g

Fats 29g

Protein 17.9g

Fiber 0.95g

Baked Manchego Chicken Wings

Serves: 4

Ingredients

20 frozen wings

1 cup of grated Manchego cheese (or Parmesan, Asagio...)

2 Tbsp Olive oil

2 tsp dried oregano

1/2 Tbs garlic powder

1 tsp garlic salt

Directions

1. Preheat oven to 450F.
2. In a baking pan greased with olive oil place frozen chicken wings. Sprinkle with salt and oregano.
3. Bake for 35 minutes.
4. Remove from oven and toss in a bowl with another tbsp of garlic oil until coated.
5. Sprinkle with grated Manchego cheese and garlic powder.
6. Serve hot.

Cooking Times

Total Time: 45 minutes

Nutritional Information

Calories 446

Net Carbs 2.6g

Fats 33g

Protein 32g

Fiber 0.68g

Baked Pork Chops in Sweet-Sour Marinade

Serves: 10

Ingredients

4.48 lbs pork chops

1 cup Apple cider vinegar

1 cup Erythritol

4 Tbs soy Sauce

1 cup Apple Cider Vinegar

1 tsp ginger

1 tsp pepper

coconut or olive oil for greasing

Directions

1. Preheat oven to 350F.
2. In a food processor, add all of the ingredients (except the pork chops).
3. Blend well to make the marinade.
4. In a greased pan place all of the pork chops and pour the marinade over it.
5. Cook for 60 minutes in a preheated oven flipping after 30 minutes.
6. Once ready place chops on a serving plate and enjoy your lunch!

Cooking Times

Preparation Time: 10 minutes

Total Time: 1 hour and 10 minutes

Nutritional Information

Calories 307

Net Carbs 11.43g

Fats 6g

Protein 45g

Fiber 0.08g

Bolognese Squash Spaghetti

Serves: 5

Ingredients

1 lb ground beef

2 1/2 cups Spaghetti squash

1 egg

3/4 cup Marinara Sauce

1 cup grated Parmesan cheese

1 cups shredded mozzarella cheese

1 tsp chili powder

1/2 tsp oregano

1/2 tsp parsley (fresh and chopped)

1/2 tsp basil

1 tsp crushed red pepper flakes

2 tsp of garlic minced

sea salt and ground fresh pepper to taste

ghee

Directions

1. Preheat oven to 350F.
2. Roast your spaghetti squash in the oven for about one hour.
3. In a saucepan, heat Marinara sauce; add oregano, parsley, basil and red pepper flakes. Cover and let simmer for a few minutes. Mix meatball ingredients in a bowl and roll into quarter-sized mini meatballs.
4. In a frying pan heat the ghee and cook meatballs covered. After 3 minutes, flip when halfway browned.
5. Once the meatballs are cooked through, transfer them into the sauce.
6. In a small bread pan, layer spaghetti squash, sauce, meatballs and mozzarella.
7. Bake on 25 for 30 minutes. Serve hot.

Cooking Times

Total Time: 45 minutes

Nutritional Information

Calories 446

Net Carbs 9.1g

Fats 30g

Protein 32g

Fiber 0.9g

Cheesy Zoodles with Fresh Basil

Serves: 3

Ingredients

2 cups zucchini noodles (zoodles)

2 Tbs fresh chopped basil

1/4 cup Pecorino Romano cheese, shaved

1/4 cup Grana Padano cheese, grated

3 Tbsp salted butter

3 cloves mashed garlic

1 tsp red pepper flakes

1 Tbsp chopped red pepper

1 Tbsp coconut oil

Salt and fresh cracked pepper to taste

Directions

1. In a frying pan over medium heat, melt butter and coconut oil. Add in garlic, chopped red pepper and red pepper flakes. Saute for 1 minute only.
2. Add in the zoodles and let cook for 1-2 minutes. Turn off heat and toss with fresh basil. Toss slightly.
3. Add in Pecorino Romano cheese and toss.
4. Finally, sprinkle on top with grated Grana Padano cheese.
5. Serve immediately.

Cooking Times

Total Time: 15 minutes

Nutritional Information

Calories 314

Net Carbs 6.1g

Fats 26g

Protein 15g

Fiber 2.3g

Spicy Spinach Casserole

Serves: 10

Ingredients

2 1/2 cups spinach, drained

2 lbs ground pork/beef

16 oz cream cheese

10 Tbsp sour cream

8 oz Emmenthal Cheese, shredded

2 cups pepper sauce

1 onion

1 red pepper

4 tsp Taco seasoning

Sliced Jalapeños to taste

Directions

1. Preheat oven to 350F. Grease one 8" square and a 9x13 baking dish.
2. Chop and sauté some jalapenos with chopped peppers and onions. Transfer to a bowl and set aside.
3. Add the spinach to the pan and cook until thawed completely. Move the spinach to the prep bowl
4. In a frying pan, add ground pork/meat and cook until browned well. Add taco seasoning and mix. Remove from fire and set aside.

5. In a bowl, add sour cream, mozzarella and cream cheese. Add in peppers, onion, spinach and ground meat.
6. Transfer this mix to prepared and greased baking dish and bake for 40 minutes.
7. Serve hot or cold.

Cooking Times

Preparation Time: 15 minutes

Cooking Time: 45 minutes

Nutritional Information

Calories 460

Net Carbs 5.3g

Fats 37g

Protein 25g

Fiber 0.8g

Cabbage with Ground Beef Stew

Serves 10

Ingredients

1 1/2 lb ground beef

2 lbs green cabbage

1/2 cup unsalted butter

1/2 cup water

3 cups pasta sauce

Salt and pepper to taste

Directions

1. In a food processor, shred quartered cabbage.
2. In a saucepan, melt the butter and add the cabbage, water and salt and pepper to taste.
3. Cover and cook for 12-15 minutes, stirring occasionally
4. In a meanwhile, in a frying pan brown the ground beefs.
5. Once browned, add the beef to the cabbage and stir well. Finally, add the pasta sauce and stir. Serve hot.

Cooking Times

Cooking Time: 15 minutes

Total Time: 25 minutes

Nutritional Information

Calories 307

Net Carbs 12.3g

Fats 22g

Protein 14.9g

Fiber 3.6g

Keto Cheese Ocean Pizza

Serves 7

Ingredients

1 lb ground beef

2 beef sausage

1 cup chopped Romaine lettuce

2 Tbs yellow onions

3 Tbs chopped dill pickle

1 1/2 cups Parmesan cheese

1/2 cup Colby cheese, shredded

1 1/2 cups Cheddar, shredded

1/4 Tbsp paprika

1/4 tsp Old Bay seasoning

1/4 tsp garlic powder

1/4 tsp onion powder

2 Tbsp organic Thousand island dressing

mustard to taste

1/4 tsp sea salt

1/4 tsp ground black pepper

olive oil

2 Tbsp water

Directions

1. In a frying pan greased with olive oil, add 1 cup Parmesan cheese evenly and then on top, 1 cup shredded Cheddar.
2. Leave to cook 2-3 minutes; use a spatula to lift the edges and underneath of the pizza, and slide out onto a flat surface. Allow to cool.
3. Repeat the same process, for the second pizza crust. Once done, set both cheese crusts aside.
4. Use a spatula and evenly spread Thousand Island dressing over the cheese crusts
5. In a frying pan add ground beef and cook until browned. Add old bay seasoning, garlic powder, onion powder paprika, 2 tbsp water, salt, ground black pepper to taste. Mix and set to simmer on low.
6. Finally, add in chopped hot dogs into slices and simmer for about 4-5 minutes.
7. Place chopped lettuce over your pizza crust.
8. In a bowl, place your pickles, onions, Colby cheese, and set aside.
9. On top of each cheese crust, add about a cup of the ground meat and hotdog mixture and spread evenly .Sprinkle with onions and pickles.
10. Drizzle mustard on top.
11. Sprinkle with more cheese if you like and serve.

Cooking Times

Total Time: 20 minutes

Nutritional Information

Calories 511

Net Carbs 2.7g

Fats 39g

Protein 33g

Chicken Angel Eggs

Serves 4

Ingredients

1 cup chicken, finely chopped

6 eggs

3 Tbs mayonnaise

1 Tbs chopped onion

1/2 tsp dill

1/2 tsp parsley

1 tsp Dijon mustard

1/2 tsp pepper mix seasoning

old bay seasoning

salt and black ground pepper to taste

Directions

1. In a bowl, mix all rest of ingredients (except eggs) until well mixed. Refrigerate the chicken salad for 10-15 minutes.
2. Boil your eggs. Shell, cool, and cut in half. Save or toss your yolks.
3. Fill your egg halves with chicken salad. Sprinkle with Old Bay or some other seasoning of your taste. Serve.

Cooking Times

Total Time: 25 minutes

Nutritional Information

Calories 161

Net Carbs 3.7g

Fats 11g

Protein 10g

Fiber 0.08g

Monterey Jack Steak

Serves 4

Ingredients

1 lb shaved steak

4 slices Monterey Jack cheese

2 Tbsp mayonnaise

1 Tbsp Dijon mustard

1/4 cup chopped green peppers

1/4 cup chopped onions

1 Tbsp minced garlic

1 Tbsp olive oil

1 Tbsp ghee

Directions

1. In a large frying pan add ghee and olive oil to warm over medium heat. Add onions, green peppers and garlic. Cook until soft, about 2-3 minutes. Add shaved steak and cook until browned several minutes.
2. Turn heat down to low. Add Dijon mustard and mayonnaise and mix.
3. Add Monterey Jack cheese on top of the steak and let melt until cheese is melted throughout, about 1 minute.
4. Serve hot.

Cooking Times

Total Time: 20 minutes

Nutritional Information

Calories 345

Net Carbs 4.3g

Fats 25g

Protein 24g

Fiber 0.4g

Pumpkin Chili

Serves 8

Ingredients

2 lbs ground beef

1 can (15 oz) pumpkin puree

1 Tbs pumpkin pie spice

3 cups 100% tomato juice

3 tomatoes, diced

1 red bell pepper

1 yellow onion

2 tsp cumin

1 Tbs chili powder

2 tsp cayenne pepper

ghee or coconut oil

Directions

1. In a large frying pan greased with ghee or coconut oil, brown the meat over medium heat.
2. Chop the onion and pepper and add into the pot with the meat. Cook 3-5 minutes or until the onions become translucent.
3. Add in the rest of the ingredients and let simmer on LOW for 30 minutes.

4. Season chili with salt and pepper to taste and cook for another 30 minutes.
5. Serve hot.

Cooking Times

Total Time: 1 hour and 20 minutes

Nutritional Information

Calories 354

Net Carbs 9.8g

Fats 25g

Protein 21g

Fiber 2.14g

Slow Cooker Roast and Chicken Stew

Serves 10

Ingredients

3 lb pot roast

1 lb chicken breast (boiled and shredded)

6 oz Italian sweet sausage

2 cups beef broth

1 cup chicken stock

1/2 medium onion (chopped)

1 can (11 oz) low carb diced tomatoes

1/4 tsp thyme

1/4 tsp celery salt

1 Tbs coconut oil

1 tsp basil

2 tsp dried dill weed

2 tsp garlic powder

2 tsp pepper

1 Tbsp garlic salt

1 tsp minced garlic

1 Tbsp oregano

1 Tbsp powdered buttermilk

4 tsp onion powder

4 tsp dried parsley

5 tsp red pepper flakes

2 tsp hot sauce

Directions

1. At the bottom of your Slow Cooker place roast, chicken breast and Italian sausages. Add on the top all other ingredients and stir lightly.
2. Close the lid and cook on LOW for about 6-8 hours.
3. Once ready, flavor to taste with some additional hot sauce, salt and pepper to your own liking and serve hot.

Nutritional Information

Calories 467

Net Carbs 3.7g

Fats 36g

Protein 30g

Fiber 1.03g

Mediterranean Pecorino Romano Breaded Cutlets

Serves 3

Ingredients

6 pork cutlets

1/2 cup grated Pecorino Romano cheese

2 Tbsp fresh lemon juice

2 Tbsp water

1 Tbsp olive oil

1 Tbsp green pepper, minced

1 Tbsp garlic, minced

salt and ground black pepper to taste

Directions

1. Heat a greasing frying pan to medium.
2. In a bowl pour water, lemon juice, olive oil, minced pepper and garlic. Season the salt and pepper to taste. Mix well.
3. In a separate bowl pour grated Pecorino Romano cheese.
4. Dip each cutlet first in liquid dressing and then in cheese.
5. Cook cutlets in pan for about 15-20 minutes. Serve hot.

Cooking Times

Total Time: 30 minutes

Nutritional Information

Calories 395

Net Carbs 2.5g

Fats 38g

Protein 9.1g

Fiber 0.16g

Oriental Garlicky Chicken Thighs

Serves 4

Ingredients

4 chicken thighs

16 whole cloves of garlic

2 Tbsp ghee

2 Tbsp juice of one fresh lemon

1 cup of baby carrots

1 onion, cut into quarters

2 tomatoes, cut in half

3 Tbsp garlic olive oil (or extra-virgin olive oil)

oregano

Salt and pepper

Directions

1. Preheat oven to 500F degrees.
2. Grease the bottom of a non-stick frying pan with garlic olive oil (or olive oil). Add in the chicken thighs together.
3. In between the thighs, wedge in the garlic gloves, onions, tomatoes and baby carrots.
4. Pour the lemon juice over the chicken thighs. Drizzle the ghee and garlic oil over the thighs.
5. Sprinkle oregano over the dish and season with salt and pepper to taste.

6. Bake in preheated oven for 25-30 minutes.
7. Reduce heat to 350 and cook for 20 minutes more.
8. Once ready, let cool for 5 minutes on a wire rack and serve hot.

Cooking Times

Total Time: 1 hour and 5 minutes

Nutritional Information

Calories 237

Net Carbs 8.9g

Fats 14g

Protein 17g

Fiber 1.3g

Pordenone Cauliflower Lasagna

Serves 10

Ingredients

12 chicken thighs

30 oz chopped cauliflower

6 green onions

1 onion, chopped

1 green pepper

6 bacon Slices

1 cup Cream Cheese

1/2 cup heavy cream

8 oz Pepper Jack Cheese, shredded

8 oz Cheddar Cheese, shredded

1 Tbsp garlic, minced

salt and pepper to taste

Directions

1. Preheat oven to350F.
2. Chop up a head of cauliflower into florets. Cook the cauliflower in the microwave on the vegetable setting. Set aside.
3. In a pan on stovetop, toss the chicken thighs with salt and pepper to taste. Add some water to about mid thigh and cook for 60 minutes. Chop up the onions and peppers and pan fry it.
4. Add all of the other ingredients, reserving 2 oz Cheddar and 2 oz of Pepper Jack Cheese.
5. Add the mixture into a large, greased casserole dish and top with the remaining cheese.
6. Cover with foil and cook for 30 minutes. Serve hot.

Cooking Times

Preparation Time: 20 minutes

Cooking Time: 1 hour and 30 minutes

Total Time: 1 hour and 50 minutes

Nutritional Information

Calories 486

Net Carbs 13,7g

Fats 35g

Protein 28g

Fiber 2.2g

Roasted Lemony Chicken & Prosciutto with Brussels sprouts

Serves 6

Ingredients

2 lbs chicken tenderloins

4 oz prosciutto

12 oz Brussels sprouts

1/2 cup chicken broth

1 1/2 cups heavy cream

1 tsp minced garlic

1 lemon, quartered and seeded

ghee or coconut oil for frying

Directions

1. Preheat oven to 400 degrees.
2. Cut the Brussels sprouts in half and boil for 5 minutes. Remove from heat and set aside.
3. In a frying pan add 1/2 cup chicken broth and bring to a boil on medium. After that, add heavy cream, minced garlic and lemon and let simmer for 5-10 minutes stirring frequently. Remove from heat and set aside.
4. In a separate frying pan, heat up some ghee and add chicken. Cook on medium high heat for several minutes, then add chopped prosciutto until chicken is cooked.

5. In a small casserole dish (9×9) and layer from bottom to top: Brussels sprouts, chicken, prosciutto, lemon cream sauce on top.
6. Bake in preheated oven for 20 minutes. Serve hot.

Cooking Times

Total Time: 40 minutes

Nutritional Information

Calories 333

Net Carbs 5.2g

Fats 16g

Protein 39g

Fiber 1.4g

Roquefort Spinach, Zoodles and Bacon Salad

Serves 5

Ingredients

4 cups of zucchini noodles

1 cup fresh broccoli

1/2 cup crumbled bacon

1 cup fresh spinach

1/3 cup Roquefort, bleu cheese, crumbled

1/3 cup bleu cheese dressing

fresh cracked pepper (to taste)

Directions

1. In a deep bowl add all the ingredients together and toss slightly with wooden spoon.
2. Serve and enjoy!

Cooking Times

Total Time: 5 minutes

Nutritional Information

Calories 81,2

Net Carbs 9,5g

Fats 3,1g

Protein 6g

Fiber 3,05g

Sour Avocado and Chicken Moussaka

Serves 8

Ingredients

8 chicken thighs, cooked

1 cup sour cream

1 cup Parmesan Cheese

4 avocados

1 onion

1 green pepper

1 Tbsp cayenne peppers sauce

salt and ground pepper to taste

coconut oil for greasing

Directions

1. Preheat oven to 350 F. Grease a baking dish with coconut oil.
2. In a pot cook your chicken thighs about 35 minutes. Peel avocados, cut in half, and slice into thin strips.
3. Line the bottom with avocado slices. In a small pan fry chopped peppers and onions until caramelized.
4. Add the chicken into a large bowl and chop it. Add remaining ingredients and mix well.
5. Spoon mixture over the avocado slices. Bake for 20 minutes.
6. Serve hot.

Cooking Times

Total Time: 35 minutes

Nutritional Information

Calories345

Net Carbs 11g

Fats 25g

Protein 20g

Fiber 6.4g

Spicy Italian Sausage and Spinach Casserole

Serves 10

Ingredients

16 oz spicy Italian sausage

2 1/2 cups frozen spinach

12 eggs

8 oz Cheddar

1 onion

9 oz Cherry Tomatoes

1 green pepper, chopped

12 Tbs Heavy Cream

Garlic powder

Onion Powder

Salt and ground pepper to taste

coconut or olive oil

Directions

1. Preheat oven to 350F. Grease casserole dish with coconut or olive oil.
2. In microwave cook the spinach. Chop the spicy Italian sausage and cook in a frying pan until browned. Remove to the big bowl and set aside.

3. In the same frying pan, cook the sliced onion and pepper. Transfer to the bowl with spinach.
4. Whisk together the eggs, spices and a heavy cream. Add the cheese to the bowl and combine, then add the egg mixture and combine.
5. Transfer to a greased casserole dish and add cherry tomatoes.
6. Cook in preheated oven for 50 minutes. Serve hot.

Cooking Times

Total Time: 1 hour and 5 minutes

Nutritional Information

Calories 343

Net Carbs 6,2g

Fats 25g

Protein 22g

Fiber 2.5g

Squash Spaghetti Lasagna Dish

Serves 14

Ingredients

2 1/2 lbs ground beef

2 large Spaghetti Squash

7 ounces whole milk Ricotta Cheese

7 ounces Mozzarella cheese, sliced

4 cups Marinara sauce

coconut or olive oil for greasing

Directions

1. Preheat oven to 375F. Grease a large baking dish with coconut or olive oil.
2. Split the Spaghetti Squash and lay face down into large glass dish and fill with water. Bake for 40-45 minutes.
3. While the Spaghetti Squash is cooking, in a large saucepan cook the ground meat and the marinara sauce. Once combined, set aside.
4. When the Spaghetti Squash is done scrap the meat of the squash to from spaghetti.
5. Assembly the lasagna in a large greased pan, start with a layer of Spaghetti Squash, then the meat sauce, then slices of mozzarella, then ricotta, then repeats until ingredients are exhausted.
6. Bake for 30-35 35 minutes until the top layer of cheese is browning. Serve hot or keep refrigerated.

Cooking Times

Total Time: 1 hour and 30 minutes

Nutritional Information

Calories 437

Net Carbs 16.4g

Fats 27,7g

Protein 28g

Fiber 1.9g

Dinner Recipes

Salmon with a Walnut Crust

Serves 2

Ingredients

Walnuts (1/2 cup)

Dijon mustard (1/2 tablespoon)

Salmon filets (6 oz.)-2

Salt

Maple syrup (2 tablespoons, sugar free)

Dill (1/4 teaspoon)

Olive oil (1 tablespoon)

Directions

1. Set oven to 350°F.
2. Put mustard, syrup and walnuts into a processor and pulse until mixture is pasty.
3. Heat oil in a pot and place the skin side down in the pan and sear for 3 minutes.
4. Top it with walnut blend and place into a lined baking dish.
5. Bake for 8 minutes.
6. Serve.

Nutritional Information

Calories 373

Net Carbs 3g

Fats 43g

Protein 20 g

Fiber 1g

Cheeseburger Casserole

Serves 6

Ingredients

Bacon (3 slices)

Cauliflower (1 ¼ cups)

Garlic powder (1/2 teaspoon)

Ketchup (2 tablespoons, no sugar)

Mayonnaise (2 tablespoons)

Cheddar cheese (4 oz.)

Ground beef (1 lb.)

Almond flour (1/2 cup)

Psyllium Husk Powder (1 tablespoon)

Onion powder (1/2 teaspoon)

Dijon mustard (1 tablespoon)

Eggs (3)

Salt

Black pepper

Directions

1. Set oven to 350 F.
2. Place cauliflower into a processor and pulse until fine like rice. Add remaining dry ingredients except cheese.
3. Add beef and bacon in processor until combined and pasty.
4. Heat skillet and cook meat for 8 minutes then add to dry ingredients in bowl along with half of cheese. Stir to combine and line a baking dish with parchment paper.
5. Press mixture into dish and top with leftover cheese. Bake for 30 minutes on top rack.
6. Take from heat, cool and slice.
7. Serve.

Nutritional Information

Calories 478
Net Carbs 3.6g
Fats 35.5g
Protein 32.2 g
Fiber 3.3g

Curried Coconut Chicken Fingers

Serves 5

Ingredients

Chicken thighs (24 oz., boneless with skin)

Pork rinds (1/2 cup, crushed)

Curry powder (2 teaspoons)

Garlic powder (1/4 teaspoon)

Salt

Black pepper

Egg (1)

Coconut (1/2 cup, shredded, unsweetened)

Coriander (1/2 teaspoon)

Onion powder (1/4 teaspoon)

For Dipping Sauce:

Sour cream (1/4 cup)

Mango extract (1 ½ teaspoons)

Garlic powder (1/2 teaspoon)

Cayenne powder (1/4 teaspoon)

Mayonnaise (1/4 cup)

Ketchup (2 tablespoons, sugar free)

Red pepper flakes (1 ½ teaspoons)

Ground ginger (1/2 teaspoon)

Liquid Stevia (7 drops)

Directions

1. Set oven to 400 F.
2. Beat egg in a bowl and slice chicken into strips.
3. Combine spices, pork rind and coconut in another bowl. Coat with egg and then in dry mix.
4. Place onto a lined baking sheet and bake for 15 minutes and turn over; bake for an additional 20 minutes.
5. Combine all ingredients for dipping sauce in a bowl and serve with chicken.

Nutritional Information

Calories 494

Net Carbs 2.1g

Fats 39.4g

Protein 29.4 g

Fiber 1.2g

Slow Cooker Lamb Curry & Spinach

Serves 5

Ingredients

Coconut or olive oil (1/3 cup)

3 copped yellow onions

4 cloves garlic , peeled and minced

2cm piece of ginger , peeled and grated

Ground cumin (2 teaspoons)

Cayenne pepper (1 1/2 teaspoons).

Ground turmeric (1 1/2 teaspoons).

Beef stock , high quality (2 cups)

Leg of lamb , cut into 2cm cubes (53 oz.)

Salt

Baby spinach (6 cups)

Plain full-fat yogurt (2 cups)

Directions

1. In a large frying pan over medium-high heat, warm oil. Add onions and garlic, and sauté until golden, about 5 minutes. Stir in ginger, cumin, cayenne, and turmeric and sauté until fragrant, or for about 30 seconds.
2. Pour in broth scraping up the browned bits on the bottom. When broth comes to a boil, remove pan from heat.

3. Put lamb in a slow cooker, and sprinkle with 1 tbsp. salt. Add contents of frying pan. Cover and cook on high-heat setting for 4 hours or low-heat setting for 8 hours.
4. Add baby spinach to pot and cook, stirring occasionally, until spinach is wilted, about 5 minutes. Just before serving, stir in 1 1/3 cups yogurt. Season to taste with salt.

Nutritional Information

Calories 304

Carbs 5.5g

Protein 32.85g

Fats 16.32g

Curried Madras Lamb

Serves 5

Ingredients

8 Fatty lamb chops

Coconut Milk (6 tablespoons)

2 cups water

Red Curry Paste (3 tablespoons)

Thai fish sauce (2 tablespoons)

Dried onion flakes (1 tablespoon)

Dried Thai or fresh red chilies (2 tablespoons)

Xylitol (1 tablespoon)

Ground cumin (1 tablespoon)

Ground coriander (1 tablespoon)

Ground cloves (1/8 teaspoon)

Ground nutmeg (1/8 teaspoon)

Ground ginger (1 tablespoon)

To Serve:

Coconut milk powder (2 tablespoons)

Red curry paste (1 tablespoons)

157

Xylitol (2 tablespoons)

1/4 cup cashews, roughly chopped

1/4 cup fresh cilantro, chopped

Directions

1. Place the raw lamb chops in a large slow cooker.
2. Add the 6 tbsp. coconut milk, water, 3 tbsp.red curry paste, fish sauce, onion flakes, chilies, 1 tbsp. Xylitol, cumin, coriander, cloves, nutmeg, and ginger. Cover and cook on high for about 5 hours (or low for 8).
3. Just before serving, scoop out the meat to another dish. Then whisk into the sauce the 2 tbsp. coconut milk powder, 1 tbsp. curry paste, 2 tbsp. sweetener, and 1/4 tsp. xanthan gum (if using).
4. Break the meat into pieces and stir into the sauce, along with the chopped cashews. Garnish with chopped coriander before serving

Nutritional Information:

Calories 190

Carbs 4g

Protein 18g

Fats 11g

Seafood Stew

Serves 5

Ingredients

Olive oil (1 tablespoon)

2 onions, diced

4 stalks celery, chopped

4 garlic cloves, minced

Dried oregano (1 teaspoon)

Ground black pepper (1/2 teaspoon)

Tomato paste (1 tablespoon)

Flour (1 tablespoon)

3 cups chicken stock

1 can tomato, onion and chili mix

1 -2 cup tomato cocktail juice

4 chicken breasts, cut into bite size pieces

2 packets mixed frozen seafood, you can add extra

mussels in at the end

2 peppers (red and green)

1 jalapeno pepper, chopped

1/4cup parsley, chopped

159

Chili powder (1 teaspoon)

1 pinch cayenne pepper

Butter (1 tablespoon)

Directions

1. In a large pan heat the olive oil and fry onions and celery
2. Add garlic, oregano, peppercorns.
3. Stir in tomato paste and almond flour and cook another minute.
4. Add chicken stock, tomatoes and tomato juice and bring to a boil. Continue to cook for about 3-5 more minutes. Remove from heat and transfer mixture to slow cooker.
5. Add chicken and stir to combine. Cover and cook on high for 3 hours or low for 6 hours.
6. Stir in mixed bags of frozen and parsley. Cover and cook on high for 30 minutes

Nutritional Information

Calories 177

Carbs 15g

Protein 21g

Fats 4g

Slow Cooker Thai Fish Curry

Serves 5

Ingredients

Coconut oil (1 tablespoon)

Green Thai curry paste (1/2 tablespoons)

8-10 spring onions

2 garlic cloves, crushed

1 Thai red chilli, deseeded if you like, and thinly sliced

Turmeric (1 teaspoon)

Chicken stock (160ml)

1½ cups coconut milk

2.5cm piece of fresh ginger, peeled and sliced

Xylitol(2 teaspoons)

Juice of 1 lime, plus extra to taste

Fish sauce(1 teaspoon)

700g boneless, skinless white fish, such as cod, hake or halibut cut into large chunks

freshly ground black pepper

chopped coriander leaves, to serve

Directions

1. Fry Spring onions, garlic and chilies then stir in green Thai Curry Paste and then sprinkle over the turmeric.
2. Add the stock, coconut milk, ginger, Xylitol and juice from a fresh lime and season with pepper. Bring to the boil, stirring to dissolve the paste and xylitol, then pour the mixture into the slow cooker.
3. Cover the cooker with the lid and cook on HIGH for 1 hour until the flavors are well blended. Add the fish sauce, if using, and add a little more xylitol and fresh lime juice, if you like.
4. Switch the cooker to LOW. Add the fish, re-cover and cook until the fish is cooked through and flakes easily..
5. Sprinkle with coriander and lime zest and sliced red chilies.

Nutritional Information

Calories 312

Carbs 20g

Protein 24g

Fats 15g

Smoky Pork Cassoulet

Serves 4

Ingredients

1 pack bacon, fried and then crumbled

Chopped onion (2 cups)

Dried thyme (1 teaspoon)

Dried rosemary (1/2 teaspoon)

3 garlic cloves, crushed

Salt (1/2 teaspoon)

Freshly ground black pepper (1/2 teaspoon)

2 cans diced tomatoes, drained

500g boneless pork loin roast, trimmed and cut into 2cm cubes

250g smoked sausage, cut into 1cm cubes

Finely shredded fresh Parmesan cheese (8 teaspoons)

Chopped fresh flat-leaf parsley (8 teaspoons)

Directions

1. Fry bacon onion, thyme, rosemary, and garlic, then add salt, pepper, and tomatoes; bring to a boil.
2. Remove from heat.
3. Place all ingredients in the slow cooker, alternating the meat with the tomato sauce until finished. Cover and cook on low for 5 hours. Sprinkle with Parmesan cheese and parsley when cooked

Nutritional Information

Calories 258

Carbs 10.8g

Protein 27g

Fats 12.6g

Sage and Orange Glazed Duck

Serves 1

Ingredients

Butter (2 tablespoons)

Swerve (1 tablespoon)

Sage (1/4 teaspoon)

Duck breast (6 oz.)

Heavy cream (1 tablespoon)

Orange extract (1/2 teaspoon)

Spinach (1 cup)

Directions

1. Use knife to score the skin of the duck and season with black pepper and salt.
2. Add Swerve and butter to a pot and cook until slightly golden then add extract and sage. Cook until butter has darkened.
3. In another pot, place chicken breast with skin side down and place over a medium flame and cook until skin is crisp.
4. Flip over and add cream to sage mixture and pour over duck. Cook until duck is done.
5. Add spinach to pot and cook until wilted.
6. Serve.

Nutritional Information

Calories 798

Net Carbs 0g

Fats 71g

Protein 36 g

Fiber 1g

Chicken Pot Pie

Serves 8

Ingredients

For filling:

Bacon (5 slices)

Garlic powder (1 teaspoon)

Cream cheese (8 oz.)

Spinach (6 cups)

Salt

Chicken thighs (6, boneless and skinless)

Onion powder (1 teaspoon)

Celery seed (3/4 teaspoon)

Cheddar cheese (4 oz.)

Chicken broth (1/4 cup)

For crust:

Psyllium Husk Powder (3 tablespoons)

Eggs (1)

Cheddar cheese (1/4 cup)

Garlic powder (1/4 teaspoon)

167

Salt

Almond flour (1/3 cup)

Butter (3 tablespoons)

Cream cheese (1/4 cup)

Paprika (1/2 teaspoon)

Onion powder (1/4 teaspoon)

Black pepper

Directions

1. Cube chicken and season with black pepper and salt.
2. Set oven to 375 °F.
3. Use spices to season chicken and place into an oven proof skillet and place onto fire and cook until golden on the outside. Add bacon to pan and cook until golden.
4. Add broth to pan along with cheeses and stir to combine. Put in spinach in pan and cook until wilted.
5. Combine dry ingredients for crust in a bowl and add cheddar and cream cheese to a microwave safe dish and then add cheese and combine. Add mixture to dry ingredients and mix together.
6. Form crust, stir ingredients in pot and top with crust and use fork to pierce crust all over.
7. Bake for 15 minutes, take from oven and cool.
8. Serve.

Nutritional Information

Calories 434

Net Carbs 3.4g

Fats 35.6g

Protein 20.4 g

Fiber 3.6g

Chicken Parmesan

Serves 4

Ingredients

For Chicken:

Chicken breasts (3)

Mozzarella cheese (1 cup)

Salt

Black pepper

For coating:

Flaxseed meal (1/4 cup)

Oregano (1 teaspoon)

Black pepper (1/2 teaspoon)

Garlic powder (1/2 teaspoon)

Egg (1)

Pork rinds (2.5 oz.)

Parmesan cheese (1/2 cup)

Salt (1/2 teaspoon)

Red pepper flakes (1/4 teaspoon)

Paprika (2 teaspoons)

Chicken broth (1 ½ teaspoons)

For Sauce:

Tomato sauce (1 cup, low carb)

Garlic (2 cloves)

Salt

Olive oil (1/2 cup)

Oregano (1/2 teaspoon)

Black pepper

Directions

1. Add flax meal, spices, pork rinds and parmesan cheese in a processor and grind until combined.
2. Pound chicken breast and whisk egg with broth in a container. Add all ingredients for sauce to a pan, stir and put over a low flame to cook.
3. Dip chicken in egg and then coat with dry mixture.
4. Heat oil in a pan and fry chicken then transfer to a casserole dish. Top with sauce and mozzarella and bake for 10 minutes.
5. Serve.

Nutritional Information

Calories 646

Net Carbs 4g

Fats 46.8g

Protein 49.3g

Fiber 2.8g

Bell Peppers Stuffed Korean Beef

Serves 4

Ingredients

Ground beef (1 lb.)

Spring onions (2, sliced)

Ginger (2 teaspoons, diced)

Eggs (8)

Bell peppers (2, cut in half)

Garlic (2 teaspoons, diced)

Salt

Black pepper

For Sauce:

Rice wine vinegar (1 ½ tablespoons)

Chili paste (1 tablespoon)

Apricot preserves (1/3 cup, sugar free)

Ketchup (1 tablespoon, low sugar)

Soy sauce (1 tablespoon)

Directions

1. Season beef with pepper and salt and start cooking over a medium flame until browned. Add ginger and garlic and stir together.
2. Push beef to one side and put in spring onions, cook for 2 minutes then stir together with beef. Take from flame and put aside.
3. Add all sauce ingredients to a pan and cook for 3 minutes then add half to beef.
4. Stir sauce and beef together and use to stuff peppers.
5. Set oven to 350 F and bake for 15 minutes.
6. Top with reserved sauce and serve.

Nutritional Information

Calories 470

Net Carbs 6.3g

Fats 35g

Protein 32.3g

Fiber 5.3g

Creamy Tarragon Chicken

Serves 1

Ingredients

Chicken breast (5 oz.)

Onion (1/4, sliced)

Chicken broth (1/2 cup)

Grain mustard (1 teaspoon)

Salt

Olive oil (1 tablespoon)

Mushrooms (3 oz.)

Heavy cream (1/4 cup)

Tarragon (1/2 teaspoon, dried)

Black pepper

Directions

1. Cube chicken and season with pepper and salt.
2. Heat oil in a pan and sauté chicken for 6 minutes until golden all over. Take from pan and put aside.
3. Add mushrooms and cook for 3 minutes until golden then add onion and cook for 3 minutes until soft and translucent.
4. Add broth and bring to a boil for 4 minutes then add remaining ingredients and adjust black pepper and salt to taste.

5. Return chicken to sauce in pan and cook for 5 minutes.
6. Serve.

Nutritional Information

Calories 490

Net Carbs 5g

Fats 40g

Protein 32 g

Fiber 1g

Beanless Chili con Carne

Serves 5

Ingredients

Ground beef (1 lb.)

Green pepper (1, chopped)

Onion (1, chopped)

Curry powder (2 tablespoons)

Cumin (2 tablespoons)

Coconut oil (1 tablespoon)

Onion powder (1 teaspoon)

Black pepper (1 teaspoon)

Italian sausage (1 lb., spicy)

Yellow pepper (1, chopped)

Tomato sauce (16 oz.)

Chili powder (2 tablespoons)

Garlic (1 tablespoon, diced)

Butter (1 tablespoon)

Salt (1 teaspoon)

Directions

1. Heat oil and butter in a pan, heat thoroughly and add garlic, onions and bell peppers. Cook for 3 minutes then add beef and sausage.
2. Cook for 5 minutes until browned then add onion and chili powder. Stir to combine and add tomato sauce. Lower flame and cook for 20 minutes.
3. Add cumin and curry, stir and cook for 45 minutes or until chili thickens to your liking.
4. Serve.

Nutritional Information

Calories 415

Net Carbs 6g

Fats 25g

Protein 146 g

Fiber 51g

Baked Cheesy Meatballs

Serves 6

Ingredients

1 lb ground beef (lean)

2 white onion

1 cup grated Cheddar cheese

4 oz Gruyere cheese

1 egg

1.5 tsp nutmeg

1.5 tsp allspice

sea salt and freshly black pepper to taste

butter for greasing

Directions

1. Preheat oven to 350F.
2. In a greased frying pan, sauté onions until translucent. Remove from heat, and let cool.
3. In a food processor mince the Gruyere cheese. Set aside.
4. In a mixing bowl, whisk egg with grated Cheddar cheese. Add the spices, salt, and pepper and mix.
5. Add in onions and Gruyere cheese. Mix well until smooth.
6. Add the beef and mix until all ingredients are combined well.
7. Divide meat mixture and roll each piece into a ball.
8. Place the meatballs on a cookie sheet, and bake in preheated oven about 20 minutes. Serve hot.

Cooking Times

Total Time: 35 minutes

Nutritional Information

Calories 385

Net Carbs 4.7g

Fats 29g

Protein 25 g

Fiber 0.9g

Chicken & Endive Casserole

Serves 6

Ingredients

1 endive head, cut into wide strips

1 1/2 lbs skinless boneless chicken thighs

1 Tbsp dried oregano

2 cups chopped onions

4 celery stalks, chopped

4 garlic cloves, chopped

1 cup diced tomatoes in juice

2 Tbsp olive oil

8 cups water

Directions

1. In a large saucepan heat oil over medium-high heat.
2. Sprinkle the chicken with salt, pepper, and oregano. Add chicken in a saucepan. Mix in onions, celery and garlic. Sauté until vegetables begin to soften, about 4-5minutes.
3. Stir in tomatoes. Add broth; bring to boil. Reduce heat to medium; simmer until vegetables and chicken are tender, about 15 minutes.
4. Add endive hearts; simmer until wilted, about 3 minutes. Season with salt and pepper.
5. Ladle into bowls and serve hot.

Cooking Times

Total Time: 40 minutes

Nutritional Information

Calories 144

Net Carbs 9g

Fats 7g

Protein 9,8 g

Fiber 2,05g

Creamy Smoked Turkey Salad with Almonds

Serves 4

Ingredients

Salad ingredients:

2 cups diced, cooked smoked turkey breast

1/4 cup sliced almonds

1/2 cup diced celery

1/4 cup sliced green onions

1/4 cup shredded cabbage

Dressing ingredients:

4 oz mayonnaise

2 oz sour cream

2 drops sweet liquid Splenda

1 tsp curry powder

Salt and pepper to taste

Directions

1. In a bowl, combine sour cream and mayonnaise and whisk until smooth. Add the spices and continue to whisk until smooth.
2. In a big bowl, combine all salad ingredients and the dressing and toss well. Serve and enjoy!

Note: *You can make the dressing a day ahead of time, and store in the fridge to let the flavors meld.*

Cooking Times

Total Time: 10 minutes

Nutritional Information

Calories 235

Net Carbs 10.9g

Fats 17g

Protein 9,8 g

Fiber 1,6g

Herb Baked Salmon Fillets

Serves 6

Ingredients

2 lbs salmon fillets

1/2 cup chopped fresh mushrooms

1/2 cup chopped green onions

4 oz butter

4 Tbsp coconut oil

1/2 cup tamari soy sauce

1 tsp minced garlic

1/4 tsp thyme

1/2 tsp rosemary

1/4 tsp tarragon

1/2 tsp ground ginger

1/2 tsp basil

1 tsp oregano leaves

Directions

1. Preheat oven to 350 degrees F. Line a large baking pan with foil.
2. Cut salmon filet in pieces. Put the salmon into the ziploc bag with the tamari sauce, sesame oil and spices sauce mixture. Refrigerate the salmon and marinade it for 4 hours.
3. Put the salmon in a baking pan and bake fillets for 10-15 minutes.
4. Melt the butter. Add the chopped fresh mushrooms and green onion to it, and mix. Remove the salmon from the oven, and

pour the butter mixture over the salmon fillets, making sure each fillet gets covered.

5. Bake for about 10 minutes more. Serve immediately.

Cooking Times

Inactive Time: 4 hours

Total Time: 35 minutes

Nutritional Information

Calories 449

Net Carbs 2,7g

Fats 34g

Protein 33g

Fiber 0,7g

Beef Cabbage Parsley Soup

Serves 8

Ingredients

1 lb beef shank

1/2 head cabbage, chopped

6 tsp fresh parsley (chopped)

2 zucchini, cubed

1 tomato, quartered

1 onion, chopped

4 cloves garlic, minced

1 Tbs salt

1/4 tsp ground cumin

2 Tbsp fresh lime juice

Directions

1.   In a large pot over low heat combine the beef, tomato, zucchini, onion, cabbage, garlic, 5 teaspoons parsley, salt and cumin.
2.   Add water to cover and stir well. Cover lid and cook for 2 hours.
3.   Remove lid, stir, and simmer for another 1 hour with lid off.
4.   Just before eating, squeeze in fresh lime juice to taste and sprinkle with remaining parsley.
5.   Serve hot.

Cooking Times

Total Time: 2 hours and 5 minutes

Nutritional Information

Calories 129

Net Carbs 13,2g

Fats 2,3g

Protein 14,1 g

Fiber 2g

Boneless Lamb Stew

Serves 6

Ingredients

2 lbs boneless lamb meat, cubed

1 cup red onion, chopped

2 whole celery stalks, diced

4 cloves garlic, minced

1 cup tomato juice

2 Tbsp extra virgin coconut oil

1 cup lime juice (freshly squeezed)

1 bay leaf

1 tsp ground cinnamon

1 tsp ground nutmeg

Fresh parsley, chopped for topping

Sea salt and freshly ground black pepper, to taste

Directions

1. Put the lamb in a glass bowl and season with the salt, pepper, cinnamon, and nutmeg. Place in refrigerator for up to 24 hours.
2. In a large casserole, heat the coconut oil over medium heat. Add pieces of lamb and brown on all sides.
3. Once browned, add the onion, garlic and celery. Cook for about five minutes, stirring often, until vegetables start to soften.
4. Add the tomato juice, lime juice and bay leaf; stir till mixture begins to boil.

5. Reduce the heat to low and cook for about 2 hours.

6. Serve hot with fresh chopped parsley.

Cooking Times

Total Time: 2 hours and 10 minutes

Nutritional Information

Calories 250

Net Carbs 6,8g

Fats 11,8g

Protein 21g

Fiber 1,6g

Keto Butternut Squash Soup

Serves 10

Ingredients

3 lbs butternut squash

4 cloves garlic, minced

1 cup yellow onion, sliced

1 cup coconut milk

2 tsp olive oil

1 bay leaf

2 cup water

1/2 tsp salt and pepper (per taste)

coconut oil or olive oil for greasing

Directions

1. Preheat oven to 450° F.
2. On a greased baking sheet, place the squash and onion with half oil and salt. Roast in a single layer about 25-30 minutes.
3. Transfer the vegetables to a large saucepan with olive oil and cook over HIGH heat for 3-5 minutes. Stir often.
4. Add garlic and cook for another 30 seconds. Add the water, bay leaf and coconut milk; bring to a boil.
5. Reduce heat to MEDIUM-LOW, cover and simmer for 10 minutes more.
6. At the end, remove bay leaf and transfer squash mixture to a blender. Puree until smooth. Add salt and pepper to taste.
7. Ladle to bowls and serve hot.

Cooking Times

Total Time: 55 minutes

Nutritional Information

Calories 120

Net Carbs 12,7g

Fats 7,2g

Protein 3,4g

Fiber 2,3g

Creamy Chicken Salad

Serves 4

Ingredients

Salad ingredients

2 cups diced, cooked chicken

1/2 cup sliced green onion

1/4 cup parsley, chopped

1/2 cup diced celery

Dressing ingredients

4 oz mayonnaise

2 oz blue cream cheese, softened

1 tsp dried tarragon

1/2 tsp dried thyme

salt and pepper to taste

Directions

1. In a bowl, whisk cream cheese and mayonnaise until smooth.
2. Add the spices and continue to whisk.
3. Combine the salad ingredients and add dressing to taste, mixing to coat all the ingredients.
4. Serve immediately.

Cooking Times

Total Time: 10 minutes

Nutritional Information

Calories 250

Net Carbs 9,7g

Fats 12g

Protein 24g

Fiber 0,7g

Duck Breast with Balsamic Vinegar

Serves 4

Ingredients

1 lb duck breasts

4 Tbsp duck fat (or lark)

4 green onions (chopped)

1 tsp fresh ginger grated

1/2 Tbsp lime juice

Marjoram to taste

2 Tbsp coconut oil

2 Tbsp apple cider vinegar

salt and freshly ground pepper to taste

Directions

1. In a frying pan add 1 tablespoon coconut oil and add the duck breast. Sauté it at high heat about 3-4 minutes.
2. In a deep saucepan add the duck fat, and add the duck meat. Cook for 3 hours about. Add the chopped green onions in the last 30 minutes of the cooking process.
3. Remove green onion and duck breast from the heat, and place them in a separate dish to cool down. Sprinkle the marjoram, balsamic vinegar and the lime juice. Serve hot.

Nutritional Information

Calories 471

Net Carbs 2,7g

Fats 46g

Protein 10g

Fiber 0,4g

Hot Mexican Meatballs

Serves 6

Ingredients

1 lb ground beef (92% lean)

4 oz white onion, minced

4 oz Monterey Jack cheese with spicy peppers

1 Tbsp butter

3 cloves garlic

1 1 tsp chili powder

1 1 tsp ground cumin

1 tsp ground coriander

1 egg

sea salt and freshly ground pepper to taste

Directions

1. Preheat oven to 350 degrees.
2. In a frying pan, sauté onions in butter until translucent. Set aside
3. Shred and mince the Monterey Jack cheese with spicy peppers. Set aside.
4. In a mixing bowl, whisk egg with ricotta cheese. Add the spices, salt, and pepper and mix.
5. Add onions and minced Monterey Jack cheese with spicy peppers. Mix well.
6. Add beef and mix until all ingredients are combined.
7. Roll the meat mix into a ball.
8. Place the meatballs on a cookie sheet, and bake about 20 minutes.

9. Serve hot.

Cooking Times

Total Time: 35 minutes

Nutritional Information

Calories 321

Net Carbs 2,9g

Fats 25g

Protein 19g

Fiber 0,9g

Lamb Cutlets with Garlic Sauce

Serves 10

Ingredients

4 lbs. lamb cutlets

1 small head of garlic, cloves peeled

2 Tbsp apple cider vinegar

1/2 cup water

1/4 cup extra virgin olive oil

pinch salt and black ground pepper to taste

Directions

1. Crush the garlic cloves thoroughly in a mortar. In a bowl, add the vinegar and water and mix it well with the crushed garlic. Set aside.
2. In a large frying pan, pour the olive oil and fry the lamb cutlets until nicely brown.
3. Add the garlic mixture and let it cook gently for about 10 minutes.
4. Shake the frying pan to spread the garlic mixture evenly over the lamb.
5. Season with salt and black pepper to taste. Serve.

Cooking Times

Total Time: 40 minutes

Nutritional Information

Calories 416

Net Carbs 0,16g

Fats 28g

Protein 36g

Fiber 0,01g

Keto Paleo Almond Bread

Serves 8

Ingredients

2 eggs

1 cup almond butter, unsalted

3/4 cup almond flour

1 Tbsp cinnamon

1 tsp pure vanilla extract

1/4 tsp baking soda

2 Tbsp liquid Stevia

1/2 tsp sea salt

Directions

1. Preheat oven to 340F degrees.
2. In a deep bowl whisk eggs, almond butter, honey, Stevia and vanilla. Add in salt, cinnamon and baking soda. Stir until all ingredients are well combined.
3. Pour dough in a greased baking pan. Bake for 12-15 minutes.
4. Once ready, let cool on a wire rack. Slice and serve.

Cooking Times

Total Time: 25 minutes

Nutritional Information

Calories 208

Net Carbs 7,6g

Fats 16g

Protein 7,7g

Fiber 3,6g

Slow Cooker Buffalo Chicken

Serves 4

Ingredients

3 Tbsp butter

6 frozen chicken breasts

1 bottle of your favorite cayenne peppers sauce

1 cup of your favorite garlic sauce

Directions

1. Put the chicken in the bottom of your Slow Cooker. Pour the hot sauce over chicken and sprinkle ranch over top

2. Cover the lid and cook on LOW for 6 hours.

3. Once ready, add butter, and cook on LOW uncovered for one hour more. Serve hot.

Cooking Times

Total Time: 6 hours and 5 minutes

Nutritional Information

Calories 517

Net Carbs 2,2g

Fats 18g

Protein 80g

Fiber 0,3g

Spiced Kale "Meatballs"

Serves 8

Ingredients

4 Tbsp olive oil

1 cup almond flour

1 bunch of kale leaves

1 green chili, chopped

1/4 tsp red chili powder

1/4 tsp turmeric powder

1 tsp cumin seed powder

1/4 tsp ginger, minced

black salt or salt as per taste

1 tsp cooking soda or baking soda (optional)

water for batter

Directions

1. In a bowl, mix all the ingredients together.
2. Combine and knead the batter with your finger. The consistency should be nor too thick nor too thin. Make a kale "meatballs".
3. Heat oil in a frying pan. Place a kale "meatballs" in the hot oil one by one.
4. Fry few at a time don't cluster with too many. When they get golden color from one side, turn and cook from another side.
5. Remove the fries with slotted spoon and place over absorbent napkins.
6. Serve hot.

Cooking Times

Total Time: 25 minutes

Nutritional Information

Calories 125

Net Carbs 13g

Fats 6,2g

Protein 6g

Fiber 4,8g

Spinach Soup with Almonds and Parmesan

Serves 6

Ingredients

1 lb baby spinach leaves

1 leek

1 zucchini (medium)

1/4 cup parmesan cheese (grated)

4 Tbsp olive oil

4 cups water

15 almond shivers

salt and black ground pepper to taste

Directions

1. Wash the leek and cut it into thick slices.
2. Heat the olive oil in a saucepan and cook the zucchini and leek for about 2-3 minutes.
3. Add the cleaned spinach leaves, water and a pinch of salt. Bring to the boil and let it simmer for 15 minutes.
4. Remove from the heat and place the vegetables in a food processor. Blend into a very smooth soup.
5. In a frying pan, toast the almonds. Pour the soup into bowls, sprinkle with some Parmesan cheese on top and toasted almonds.
6. Serve.

Cooking Times

Total Time: 45 minutes

Nutritional Information

Calories 63,4

Net Carbs 5,9g

Fats 3,04g

Protein 4,84g

Fiber 2,4g

Stuffed Avocado with Tuna

Serves: 4

Ingredients

2 ripe avocados, halved and pitted

1 can (15 oz) solid white tuna packed in water, drained

2 Tbsp mayonnaise

3 green onions, thinly sliced

1 Tbsp cayenne paprika

1 red bell pepper, chopped

1 Tbsp balsamic vinegar

1 pinch garlic salt and black pepper to taste

Directions

1. In a bowl, toss together tuna, mayonnaise, cayenne pepper, green onions, red pepper, and balsamic vinegar.
2. Season with pepper and salt, and then pack the avocado halves with the tuna mixture.
3. Ready! Serve and enjoy!

Cooking Times

Total Time: 20 minutes

Nutritional Information:

Calories 233,3

Net Carbs 9,69g

Fats 17,77g

Protein 7,41g

Fiber 6,98g

Keto Light Cabbage Soup

Serves: 4

Ingredients

2 1/2 cups chopped cabbage

4 garlic cloves, minced

1 Tbsp tomato paste

1 onion, chopped

1/2 cup parsnip, chopped

1/2 cup cauliflower florets

1/2 cup chopped zucchini

1/2 tsp basil

1/2 tsp oregano

Salt and black pepper, to taste

4 cups water

olive oil for sautéing

Directions

1. In a frying pan, sauté onions, parsnip and garlic for 5 minutes.
2. Add in water, tomato paste, cabbage, cauliflower, basil, oregano and salt and pepper to taste.
3. Simmer for a about 5-10 minutes until all vegetables are tender. Add the zucchini and simmer for another 5 minutes.
4. Serve hot.

Cooking Times

Total Time: 35 minutes

Nutritional Information

Calories 80,31

Net Carbs 9,69g

Fats 3,08g

Protein 4,62g

Fiber 1,6g

Oriental Shrimp Soup

Serves: 8

Ingredients

12 oz fresh shrimp, peeled and deveined

1 cup zucchini (medium, sliced)

1 onion, chopped

2 cloves garlic, minced

1 Tbsp ginger, minced

1 pinch crushed red pepper

2 quarts water

1 cup celery (chopped)

2 cups cauliflower florets

2 Tbsp soy sauce

1/4 tsp ground black pepper

2 tsp olive oil

Directions

1. In a large saucepan with over medium heat cook onion, garlic, ginger and crushed red pepper for 2 minutes.
2. Pour in water, cauliflower florets and celery and bring to a boil. Reduce heat, cover and simmer 5 minutes.
3. Stir in zucchini and shrimp, season with salt and pepper to taste; cover and cook 5 - 7 minutes.

4.   Stir in soy sauce and pepper and serve.

Cooking Times

Total Time: 25 minutes

Nutritional Information:

Calories 107,62

Net Carbs 7,12g

Fats 3,08g

Protein 12,08g

Fiber 1,6g

Slow Cooker Beef with Dried Herbs

Ingredients

1 1/2 lbs lean beef

2 celery ribs

1 cup beef broth

2 Tbsp amaranth flour

2 Tbsp almond butter

2 Tbsp olive oil

1 tsp mustard

2 Tbsp fresh lemon juice

4 Tbsp chopped parsley

salt, pepper, dried thyme, dried marjoram

Directions

1. In a bowl, toss the beef with the amaranth flour. Heat the butter and oil in a skillet; add the beef and cook, stirring, until browned.
2. In a slow cooker combine the browned beef with remaining ingredients, except lemon juice and parsley.
3. Cover and cook on LOW for 6 to 8 hours.
4. Once ready, stir in lemon juice and parsley and serve hot.

Nutritional Information:

Calories 387,96

Net Carbs 2,56g

Fats 12,53g

Protein 20,96g

Fiber 0,2g

Zucchini Soup with Crunchy Cured Ham

Serves 4

Ingredients

2 leeks (white part only)

12 ounces zucchinis

10 ounces summer squash

3 Tbsp virgin olive oil

5 cups water

salt

2 slices cured ham

black pepper

Directions:

1. Cut the leeks into thin slices and chop the zucchinis and summer squash into cubes.

2. In a large saucepan, heat the olive oil and add the leeks. Cook the leeks until they are soft, stirring gently.

3. Add in the chopped zucchinis and summer squash and cook them for about 5 minutes.

4. Add in water and bring to the boil for about 15 minutes.

5. Blend or process the soup in batches until smooth.

6. Season the soup to taste.

7. In a frying pan cook striped ham until crispy.

8. Divide the soup amongst the serving bowls and sprinkle with the crunchy ham strips and some black pepper.

9. Serve hot.

Cooking Times

Total Time: 45 minutes

Nutritional Information

Calories 84,19

Net Carbs 8,75g

Fats 31.7g

Protein 8,54g

Fiber 1,52g

Seared Ribeye Steak

Serves 3

Ingredients

Ribeye steaks (2 medium)

Salt

Black pepper

Bacon fat (3 tablespoons)

Directions

1. Set oven to 250 F.

2. Place a wire rack over a baking sheet and place steaks on rack.

3. Use pepper and salt to season steaks and bake until steak's internal temperature is 123 F.

4. Melt fat in a cast iron pan until it is extremely hot then transfer steaks to pot and sear on both sides.

5. Let steaks sit for a few minutes before slicing.

6. Serve.

Nutritional Information

Calories 430

Net Carbs 0g

Fats 31.7g

Protein 30.3 g

Fiber 0g

Snacks

Greek-Style Fat Bomb Balls

Serves: 5
Serving Size: 1 ball

Ingredients

Cream cheese, softened (1/2 cup)

Butter, softened (1/4 cup)

Freshly chopped or dry herbs (3 teaspoons) - (any combination of basil, thyme, oregano and/or parsley works great) 4 pieces sun-dried tomatoes, drained

4 Kalamata olives, pitted and chopped

2 cloves garlic, crushed

freshly ground black pepper

Sea salt (1/4 teaspoons)

Parmesan cheese, finely grated (5 tablespoons)

Directions

1. Mash the butter and cream cheese together with a fork and mix until well combined. Mix in the chopped sun-dried tomatoes and chopped Kalamata olives.
2. Add the freshly chopped herbs (or dried), crushed garlic and season with salt and pepper. Mix well and place in the fridge for 20-30 minutes to firm up.
3. Remove the cheese mixture from the fridge and start creating 5 balls. A spoon or an ice-cream scooper works well.

4. Place the grated parmesan cheese in a shallow dish. Roll each ball in the grated parmesan cheese and place on a plate. Eat immediately or store in the fridge in an airtight container for up to a week.
5. Enjoy!

Nutritional Information

Calories: 164

Fat: 17.1

Bacon & Onion Cookie Bites

Serves: 12

Serving Size: 1 cookie

Ingredients

Almond flour (1 ½ cups)

Flax meal (1/3 cup)

Psyllium husk powder (1 tablespoon)

Onion powder (1 tablespoon)

1 large egg

4 slices bacon, cooked until crispy and crumbled

Sea salt (1/2 teaspoon)

Freshly ground pepper

Directions

1. Place all of the dry ingredients into a bowl (almond flour, flax meal, psyllium husk powder, onion powder, salt and pepper) and mix until well combined.

2. If you don't have onion powder, you can use dried onion flakes and blend them until powdered. Also, make sure you don't use whole psyllium husks - blend the psyllium husks until powdered if needed.

3. Add the egg and mix well using your hands.

4. Add the crumbled bacon to the dough. Process well using your hands. (Be sure to save the bacon fat from the cooking process for other uses - like some of the other fat bomb recipes in this book.)

5. Using your hand, create 12 equal balls and place them on a baking sheet lined with parchment paper.

6. Use a fork to press and flatten the dough.

7. Transfer into the oven and bake for 10-12 minutes. Keep an eye on the cookies. Almond flour can burn easily and cause the cookies to taste bitter. When done, the cookies should be golden brown. Remove from oven and cool on a wire rack.

8. Store at room temperature covered with a kitchen towel or in a container.

9. Enjoy!

Nutritional Information

Calories: 109

Fat: 9

Guacamole & Bacon Fat Bombs

Serves: 6

Serving Size: 1 fat bomb

Ingredients

1 large avocado

Butter, softened (1/4 cups)

2 cloves garlic, crushed

Crushed red pepper (1 teaspoon)

½ small white onion, diced

Fresh lime juice (1 tablespoon)

Freshly ground black pepper

Sea salt (¼ teaspoon)

4 large slices bacon

Bacon grease, reserved from cooking (2 tablespoons)

Directions

1. Preheat the oven to 375 Fahrenheit. Line a baking tray with parchment paper. Lay the bacon strips out flat on the parchment paper, leaving space so they don't overlap. Place the tray in the oven and cook for about 10-15 minutes until golden brown and crisp. The time will depend on the thickness of the bacon slices. When done, remove from the oven and set aside to cool down.

2. Halve, deseed and peel the avocado. Place the avocado, butter, crushed red pepper, crushed garlic and lime juice into a bowl and season with salt and pepper.

3. Mash using a potato masher or a fork until well combined. Add the diced onion and mix well.

4.   Pour in the 2 tablespoons of reserved bacon grease and mix well. Cover with foil and place in the fridge for 20-30 minutes to firm up.
5.   Chop the bacon into small pieces and place in a shallow dish.
6.   Remove the guacamole mixture from the fridge and start creating 6 balls. You can use a spoon or an ice-cream scooper. Roll each ball in the bacon crumbles and place on a tray that will fit in the fridge.
7.   Eat immediately or store in the fridge in an airtight container for up to 5 days.

Nutritional Information

Calories: 156

Fat: 15.2

Bacon and Egg Fat Bombs

Serves: 6
Serving Size: 1 ball

Ingredients

2 large eggs

Butter, softened (¼ cup)

Mayonnaise (2 tablespoons)

Freshly ground black pepper

Sea salt (1/2 teaspoon)

4 large slices bacon

Bacon grease, reserved from cooking (2 tablespoons)

Directions

1. Preheat the oven to 375 Fahrenheit. Line a baking tray with parchment paper. Lay the bacon strips out flat on the baking paper, leaving space so they don't overlap. Place the tray in the oven and cook for about 10-15 minutes until golden brown and crisp. The time depends on the thickness of the bacon slices. When done, remove from the oven and set aside to cool down.

2. Hard boil the eggs. Fill a small saucepan about three quarters of the way with water. Add a good pinch of salt. This will help to prevent the eggs from cracking. Bring the water to a boil. Using a spoon or your hand, carefully dip each egg into the boiling water - be careful not to burn yourself. Cover the saucepan and turn off the heat. Set a timer for 10 minutes. When 10 minutes is up, rinse the eggs under cold water to stop the cooking process.

3. Peel and quarter the hard boiled eggs.

4. Cut the butter into small pieces and add the peeled and quartered eggs. Mash with a fork.

5. Add the mayonnaise, season with salt and pepper and mix well. Pour in the bacon grease and combine well. Place in the fridge for 20-30 minutes or until firm and easy to form fat bombs.

6. Chop the bacon into small pieces and place in a shallow dish. Remove the egg mixture from the fridge and roll out 6 balls. You can use a spoon or an ice-cream scooper. Roll each ball in the bacon crumbles and place on a tray that will fit in the fridge.

7. Eat immediately or store in the fridge in an airtight container for up to 5 days.

Nutritional Information

Calories: 185

Fat: 18.4

Simple Parmesan Crisps

Serves: 4

Serving Size: 5 crisps

Ingredients

Parmesan cheese (1 cup)

Coconut flour (4 tablespoons)

Rosemary, oregano or any herbs of choice, dried or fresh (1-2 teaspoons)

Directions

1. Preheat the oven to 350 Fahrenheit. In a small bowl, mix the coconut flour and grated parmesan cheese. Don't use finely grated, or powdery parmesan cheese like you find in a canister at the supermarket, as it won't work well in this recipe. Try to find finely grated parmesan in the deli section of your supermarket, or even better, grate your own!

2. You can add any herbs you like. Oregano and rosemary work wonderfully.

3. Scoop a teaspoon of the cheese mixture onto a baking tray lined with parchment paper leaving a small gap between each. Place in the oven and cook for 10-15 minutes or until golden brown, but be careful not to burn.

4. Remove from the oven and let the crisps cool down before you remove them from the baking tray.

5. Enjoy!

Nutritional Information

Calories: 233

Fat: 14.5

Conclusion

Thank you again for purchasing this book!

I certainly hope this book has gotten you ready to take on the ketogenic journey. I am more than happy that you have decided to take control of your health. Many of us are facing a deep food problem that is making our lives miserable and that is slowing us down. No longer will you sit back and watch your life slip on by. You are now more than equipped with all the arsenal to fight off your unhealthy habits in favor of a clean, healthy and vibrant life.

The next step is to get into the program so you can have firsthand experience of all the benefits we have spoken about in this book. Most importantly, we want you to take part. We need you to take this seriously and see all the amazing results in even unexpected areas.

Even if you don't believe that the Ketogenic diet will make a significant change in your life, what would it hurt to give it a try? If you are willing to sacrifice 30 short days to make yourself better from the inside out with guaranteed results, isn't it worth it? Just do it! It's that important and we trust in it that much!

The Ketogenic diet has changed our lives and we want it to change and improve your life as well! Say hello to a renewed you!

Finally, if you feel that you have received any value from this book, then I'd like to ask if you would be kind enough to click on the link below and leave a review on Amazon to share your positive experience with other readers.

It'd be greatly appreciated!

Before you go, be sure to flip to the next page to see some of my other books which you may be interested in...

counseling. The information presented herein has not been evaluated by the U.S Food & Drug Administration, and it is not intended to diagnose, treat, cure or prevent any disease. Full medical clearance from a licensed physician should be obtained before beginning or modifying any diet, exercise or lifestyle program, and physician should be informed of all nutritional changes. The author claims no responsibility to any person or entity for any liability, loss or damage caused or alleged to be caused directly or indirectly as a result of the use, application or interpretation of the information presented herein.

CPSIA information can be obtained at www.ICGtesting.com
Printed in the USA
LVOW07s0603080716

495488LV00035B/502/P